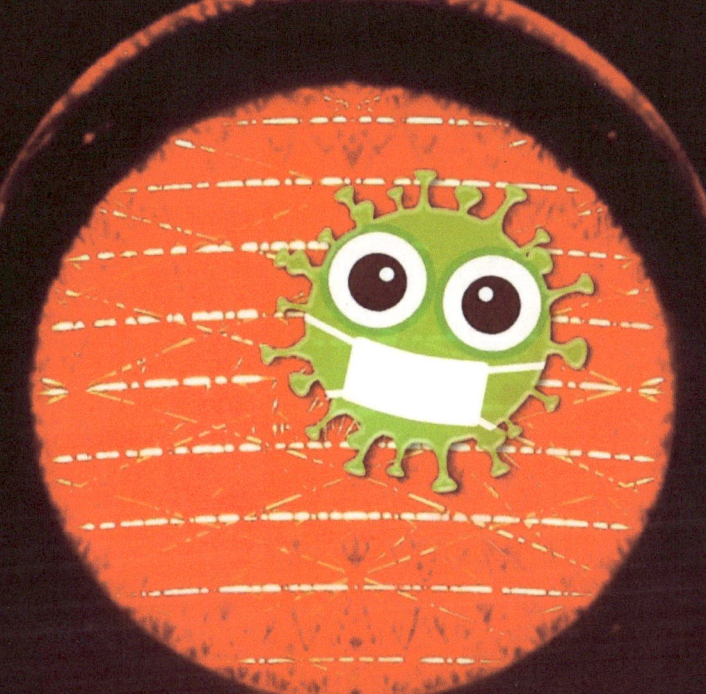

Linda Mason

THE COVID-19 MONSTER

A "Spirit of Truth" Storybook

Copyright Page

The COVID-19 MONSTER

A "Spirit of Truth" Storybook

Published by: Books By L Mason "A Safe Place"
Author: Linda Mason
Editor: Tamara Mason
Cover Design: SelfPubBookCovers.com/BravoCovers

P.O. Box 1162
Powhatan, VA 23139
www.BooksbyLMason.com
LMasonOnTop@aol.com
ISBN: 9798643427360
© 2020 by Linda C Mason
WGA West Registration: 2071205

All Rights Reserved

No part of this book, including contents or cover, may be reproduced in whole or in part without the expressed written consent of the author. **You have my permission to copy the symptoms worksheet on page 63.**

Printed in the United States of America

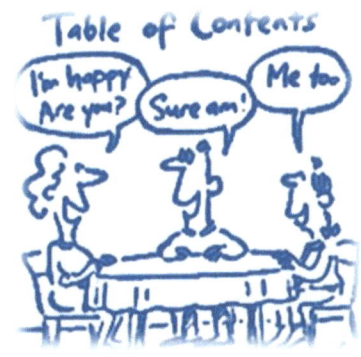

Dedication page and Introduction	4
Introduction	5
Part 1: The Virus	6
Part 2: The Child	24
Part 3: Tellin' It Like Some Perceive It to Be	43

    Affection During This Time of COVID-19
    Religion During This Time of COVID-19
    Protected Commodities During This Time of COVID-19
    Shopping During This Time of COVID-19
    Quarantining During This Time of COVID-19
    Fake News and Hypocrisy During This Time of COVID-19
    Testing During This Time of COVID-19
    Mixed Messaging During This Time of COVID-19
    Political Propaganda During This Time of COVID-19
    Misguided Youth Thinking During This Time of COVID-19
    How Will YOU Respond to COVID-19?
    Never Forget Our Heroes

Prevention	58
What about My Pets?	59
Note to parents	61
Child Symptoms of COVID-19 worksheet	70
Child Symptoms of COVID-19 answer sheet	71
Other publications	72
About the Author	75

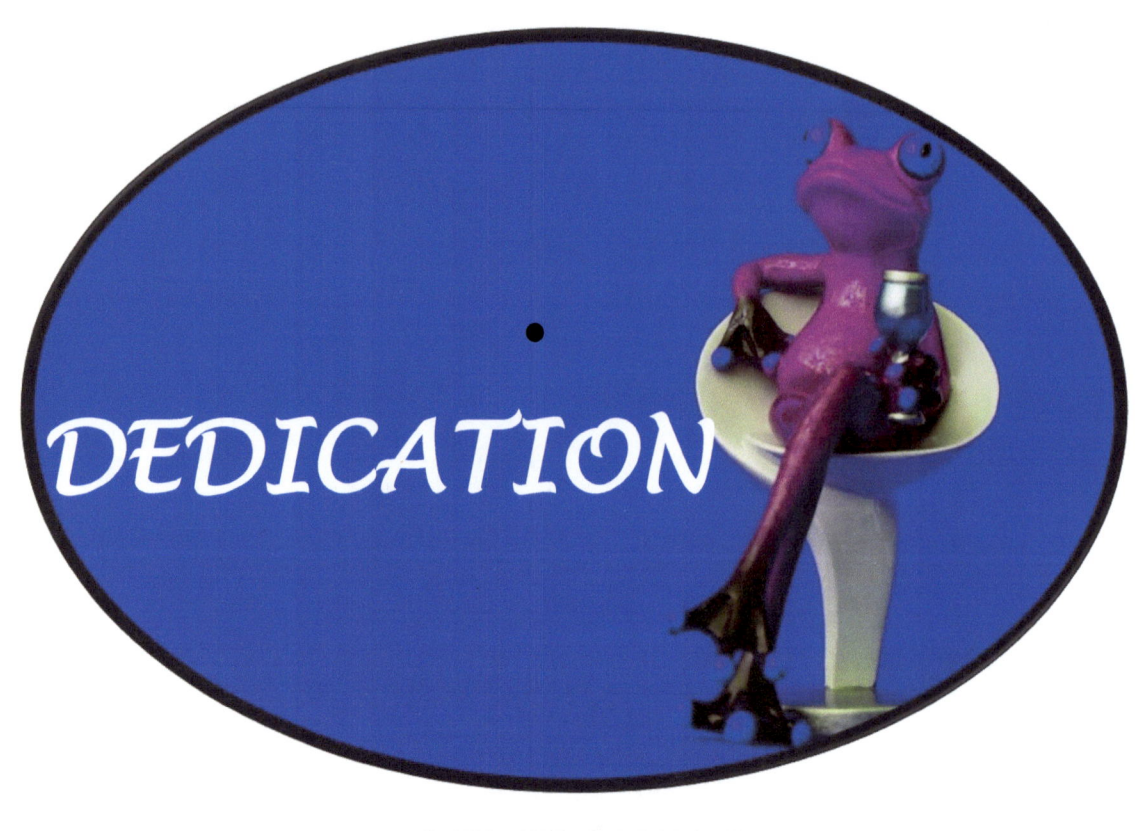

DEDICATION

I dedicate this book to my three grandchildren, who may be wondering what this terrible invisible virus is all about. Niyah, Laana, and Aaron, along with the rest of my supportive family, are the heartbeat of my survival. With the grace and strength of Jesus Christ, May all of you fulfill your appointed days and assigned destinies.

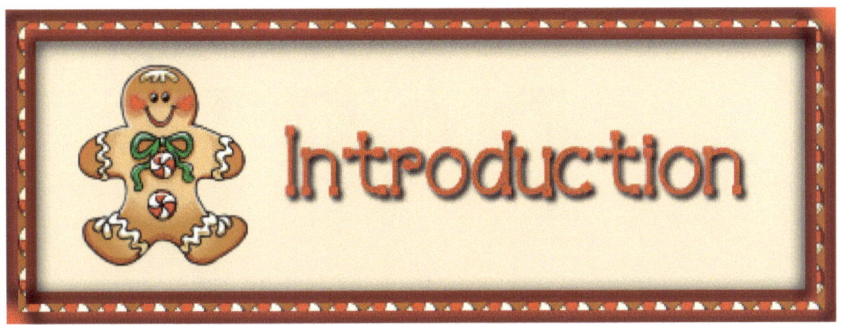

Introduction

This book was written to help provide information in an age-appropriate manner about the Coronavirus pandemic spreading rapidly throughout our world today (2020). Having three young grandchildren, I felt that they would be able to face this monster with less fear if they knew how it came to be and if they could help in any way. This storybook was designed with children in mind; its pages are overflowing with vivid color and bubbly illustrations that make it irresistible to the average youngster. Even though children can understand the book as young as four or five years old, it can be read by fourth-graders or above. Adults can be enriched through the valuable information provided as well, including information on animal/human spread of this virus and current scientific statistics. Check out *Note to parents* on page 57.

This storybook includes a unique interactive bonus, as do many of my other *Spirit of Truth Storybooks* — a secret coded message scattered throughout this book highlighted in red lettering. These letters spell out children's symptoms of the condition recently discovered by doctors that seem to be linked to COVID-19. A worksheet to record these letters has been provided for your child's enrichment and curiosity as they move through the book and discover the named symptoms.

A portion of the proceeds from the sale of this book will be donated to a memorial fund for families who have lost children to this invisible Coronavirus enemy. Will you help make it count?

PART

1

The Virus

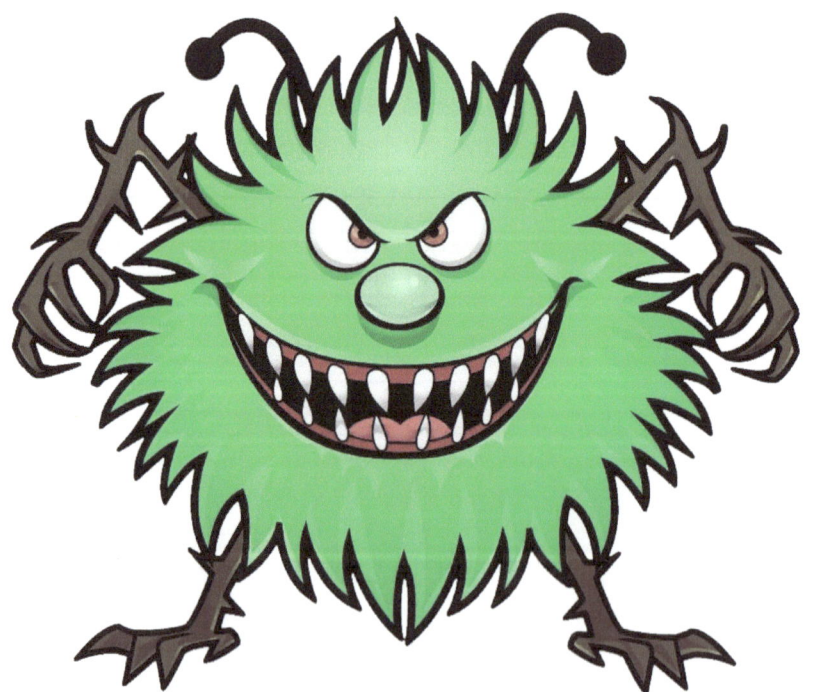

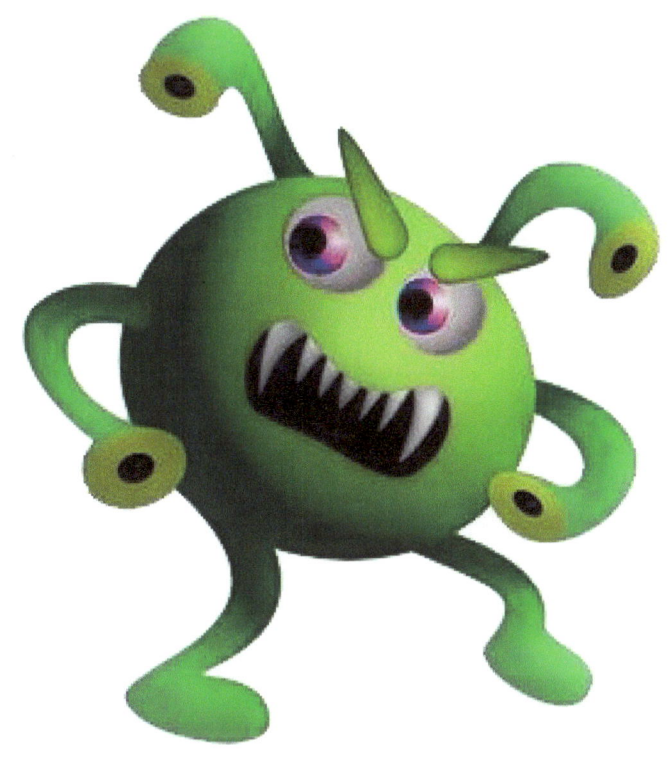

Hi, my name is COVID-19. Some people call me the novel Coronavirus, but you can call me *Dangerous*. I'm a close cousin to the flu but can do a lot more damage.

Doctors have finally realized that children ages 10 and above can spread me equally as fast as their parents. Children can have various symptoms like fevers with a rash, red or pink itchy eyes, stomach pains, diarrhea, and vomiting, all within four

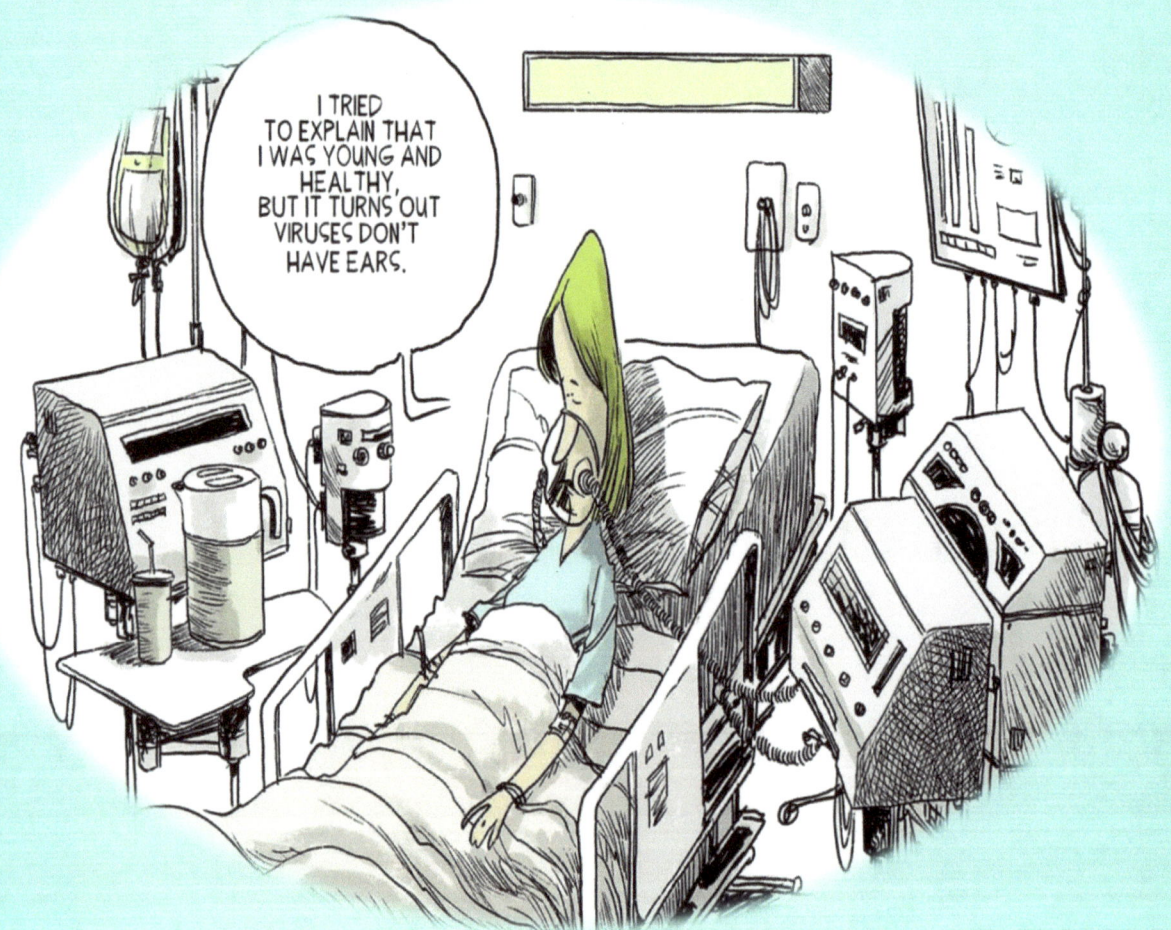

Dave Granlund-Editorial Cartoons and Illustrations, davegranlund.com

days of contracting me. They may also have no symptoms at all. Pretty cool, huh?

I love to travel. I jump from hand to hand through **high fives** and **handshakes**. I can move from person to person through **cough droplets** and **sneezes**, too.

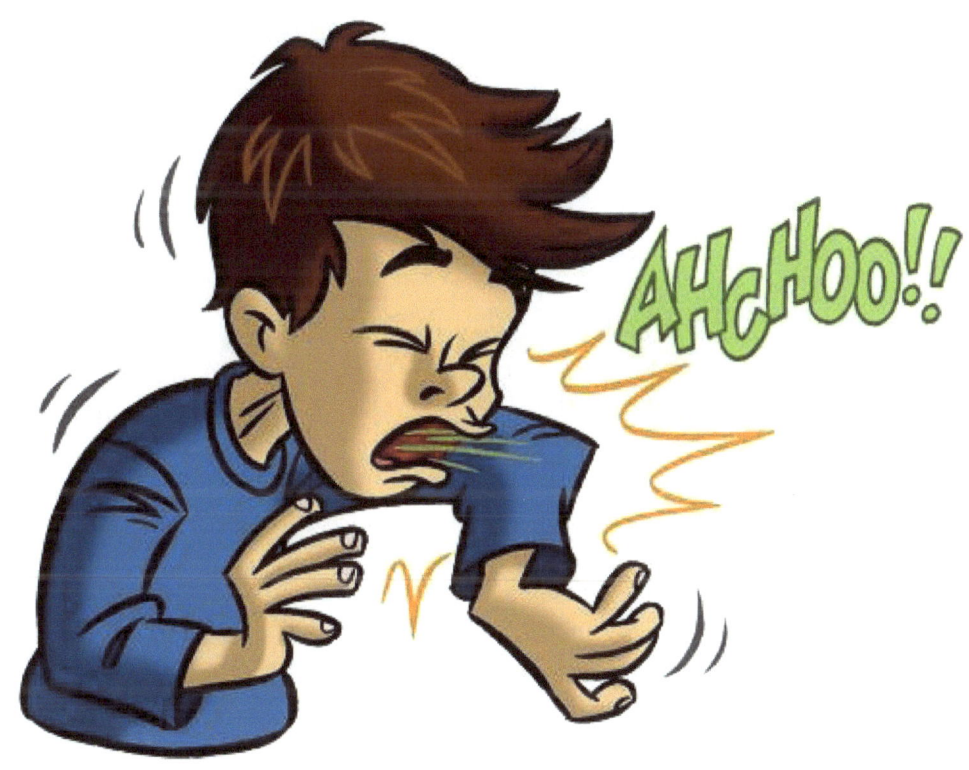

Sometimes, I leave the people with "COVID toes" once they test positive and over time, they test negative again. It's one of the many aftereffects, you know. I want them

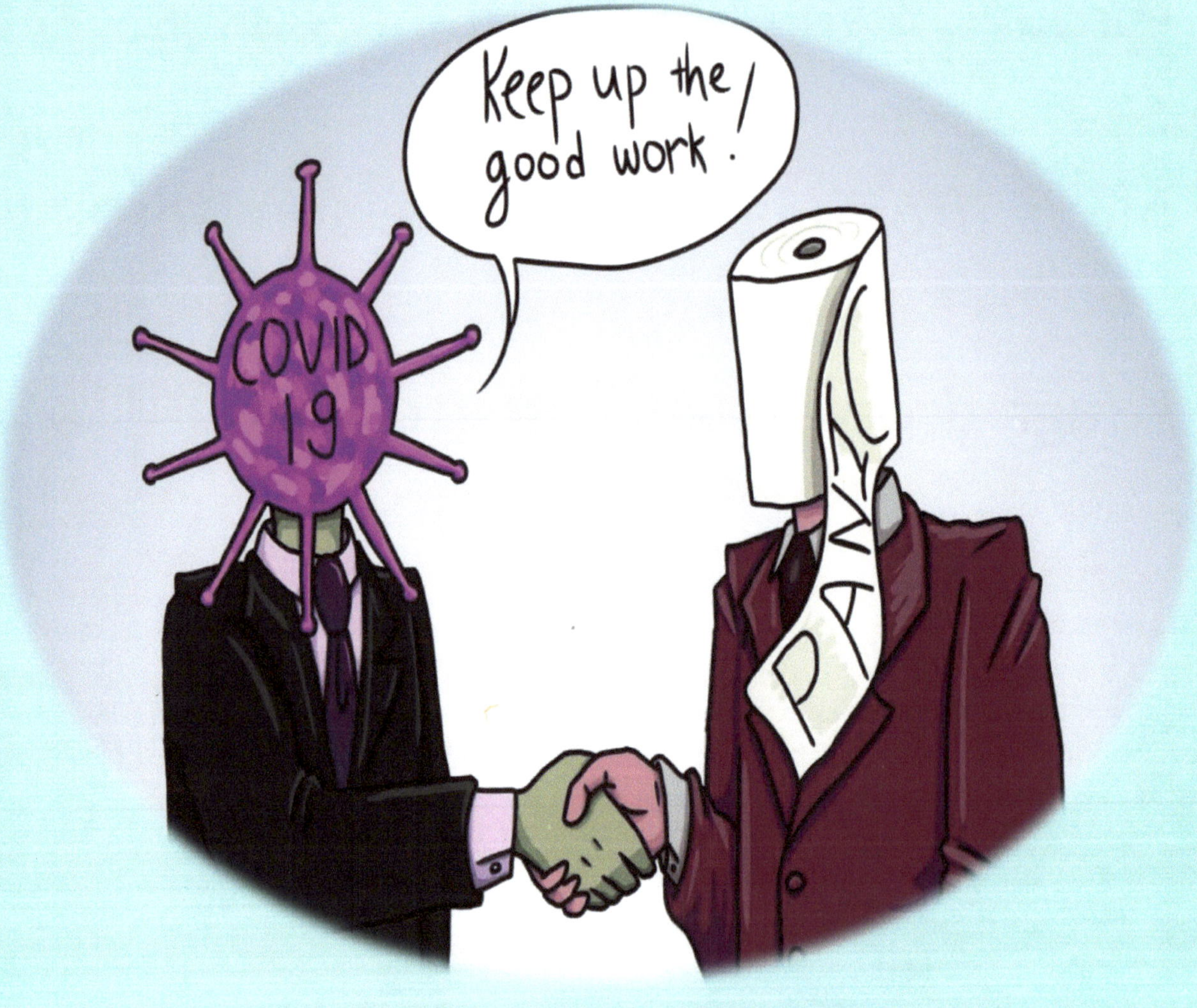

COVID-19 Meets Panic-Scot Scoop News, scotscoop.com

to remember me.[1]

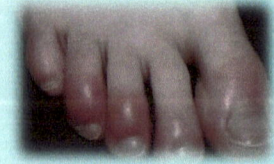

Oh, I'm very sneaky and invisible, too. You can't even see me coming. If you stand close to someone not wearing a mask and they just breathe, I can still jump from them to you *soooo* easily. Ha, ha, ha! High five that!

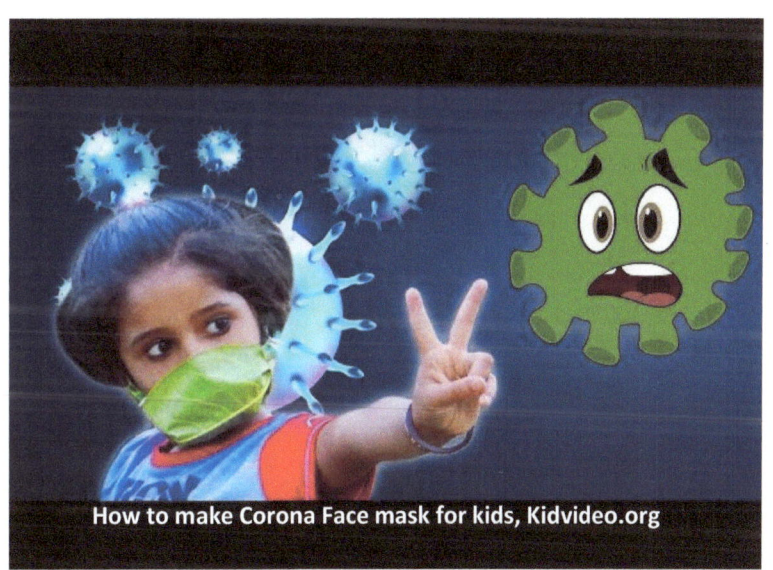

I can travel from state to state in a very short time, and from country to country just as fast. I don't stay long in the bodies of those I **c**hoose to visit, and everyone I invade gets better... well, almost everyone. Cool, **h**uh?

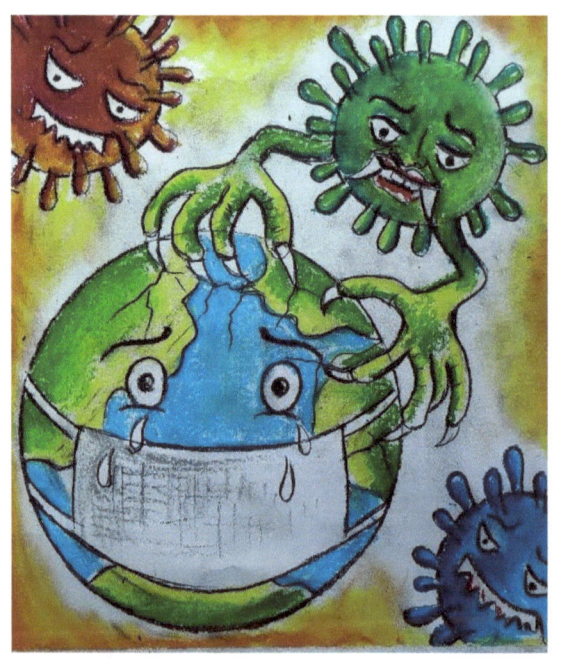

How to draw Coronavirus /drawing of earth
from www.youtube.com

When I come to visit, I'm usually not welcomed, but that doesn't bother me. I jump right into their bodies and get to work, making them feel bad very quickly. I'm excellent at what I do. Do you know anyone who wants to hire me? I work for FREE!

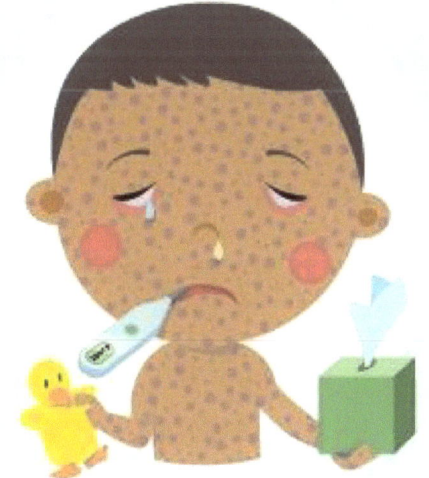

You see, I also bring some very hard working virus buddies with m**e** that cause coughs, bod**y** aches, sore throats, fevers, h**e**adaches, shortness of breath, and even a loss of smell or taste, so you won't be able to enjoy yummy food**s** for a while. They work for FREE, too.

I'm a very cunning virus and most people, even adults, are extremely afraid of me. And do you know what? They should be because I'm a nasty, horrible monster!

Remember, I don't usually stay very long, maybe a week or two, but sometimes I

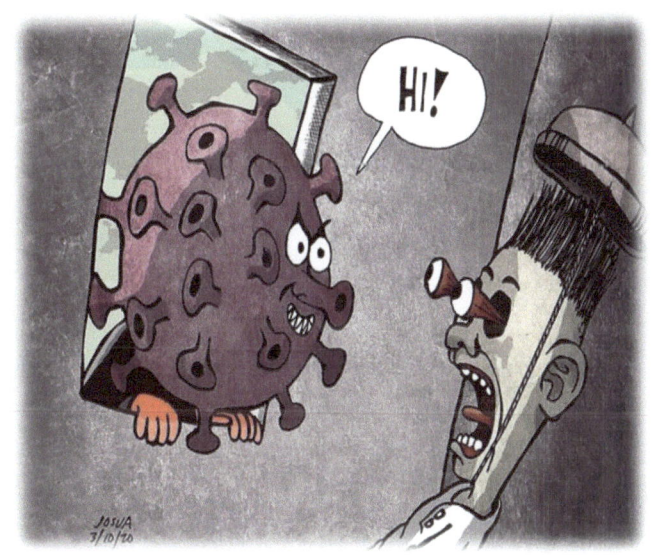

Editorial Method vs COVID-19, YAHOO!

decide to **s**tick around for one or more

months.

The choice is mine. Don't tell anyone, but

most people can get rid of me or even

keep me from visiting them altoget**h**er by

practicing 'physical

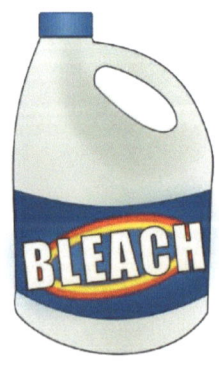
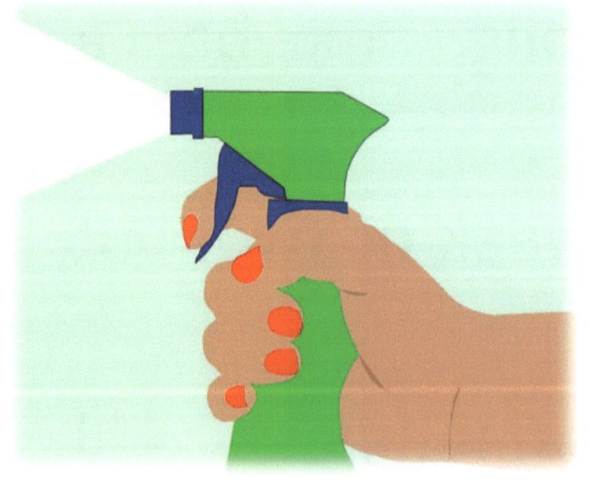

distancing' and keeping everything, especially their hands, washed several times a day. **S**oaps and disinfectants are not my friends.

I run away when they use **t**hose things, but I can come back when they get dirty again. That is why I just hate it when 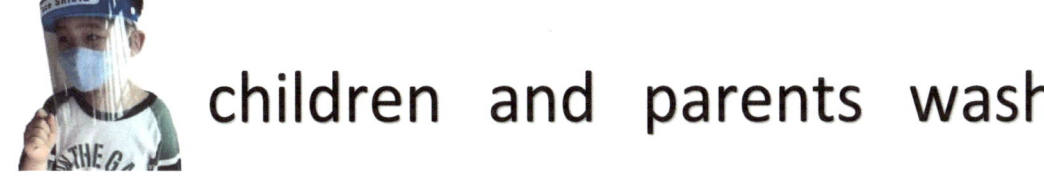 children and parents wash their

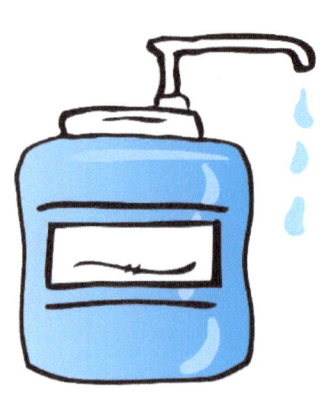 hands over and over again, wear masks or face shields in pubic, and practices physical distancing while I'm in town with my viral buddies. It's not fair!

Physical distancing, 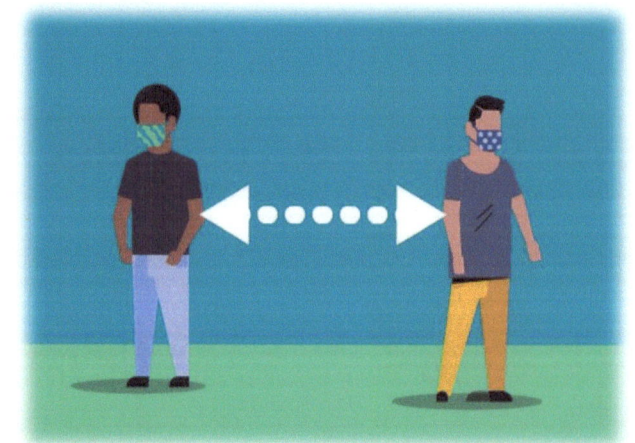 sometimes called "social distancing," is when you wear face masks and stay far apart from other people and children when you leave your homes to go to the grocery store or other pla**c**es.

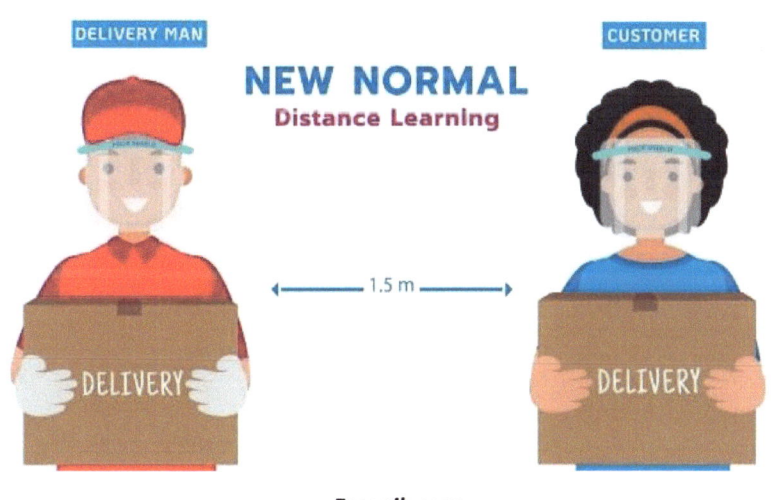

I can't jump on people when they are

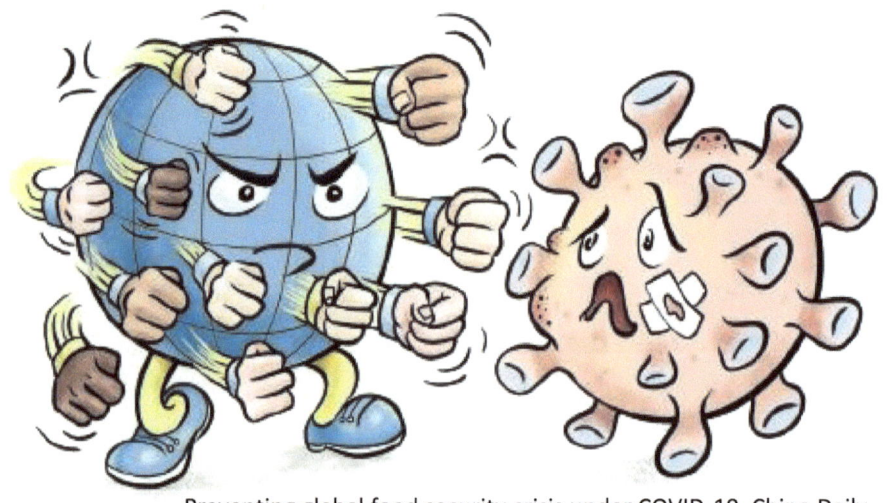
Preventing global food security crisis under COVID-19, China Daily

protected and far away from each other.

When I can't jump on people and make

them sick, they are much happier, but I'm

mad. You see, it's my job to make them

miserable! So I guess if they keep using soap and water and disinfectants and continue to practice physical distancing until a vaccine is developed, they will always stay safe from me. Phooey! I hope they are slow to make a vaccine. A vaccine is a medicine that the scientist and doctors develop that keeps my buddies and me from getting into human bodie**s** and making them sick. What am I going to do with all my time if I can't make them sick? It can take many months for **d**octors to create a vaccine or find a cure, but until then, my buddies and myself will

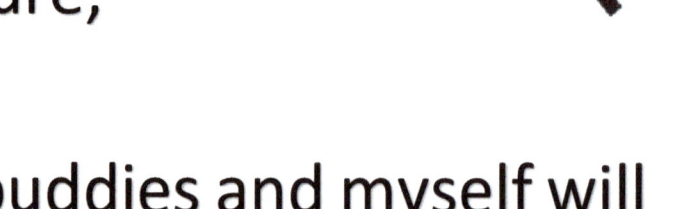

continue to have a party at your expense-

- unless you wash us away with that soap

and water and those awful dis**i**nfectants.

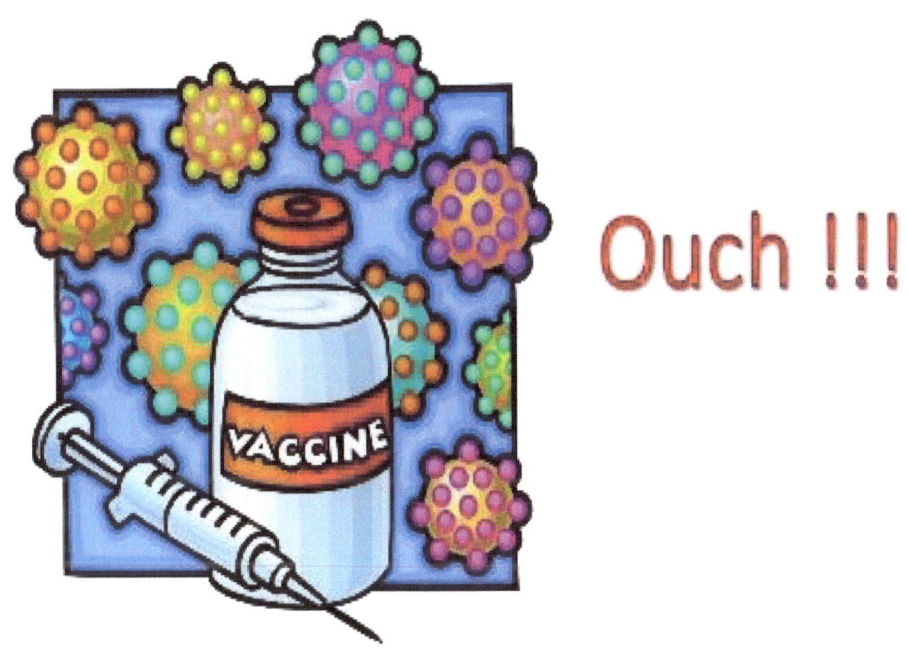

Ouch !!!

PART 2

The Child

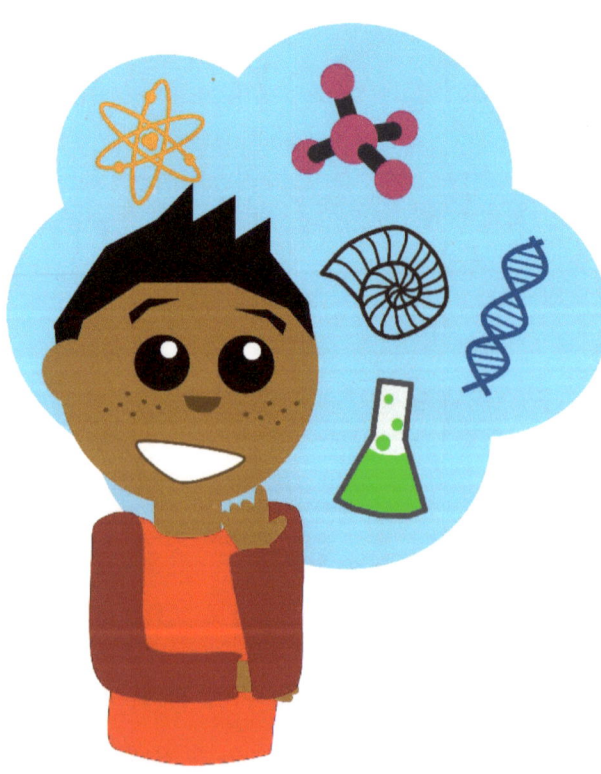

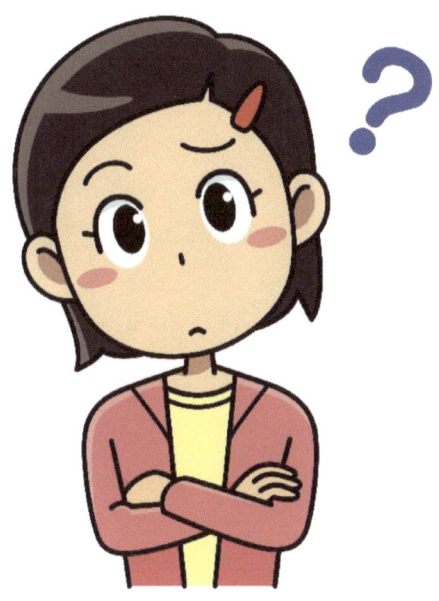

I w**a**nna go to the Children's Museum and other places to get outside.

But the COVID-19 monster may be lurking around and will su**r**ely get inside.

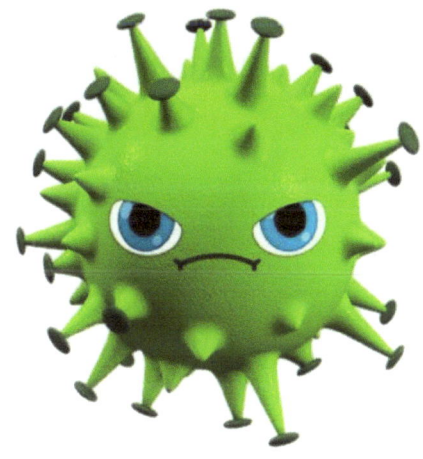

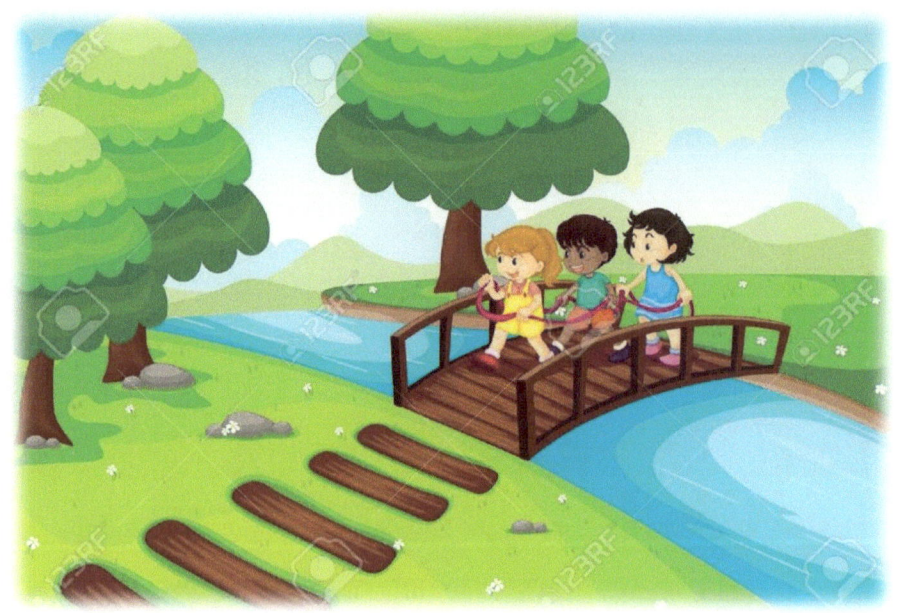

I wanna go to the zoo and

to the playgrounds at the park,

But the COVID-19 monster is out there

and has dulled my happy spark.

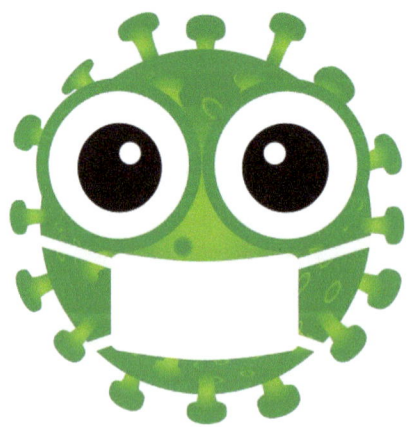

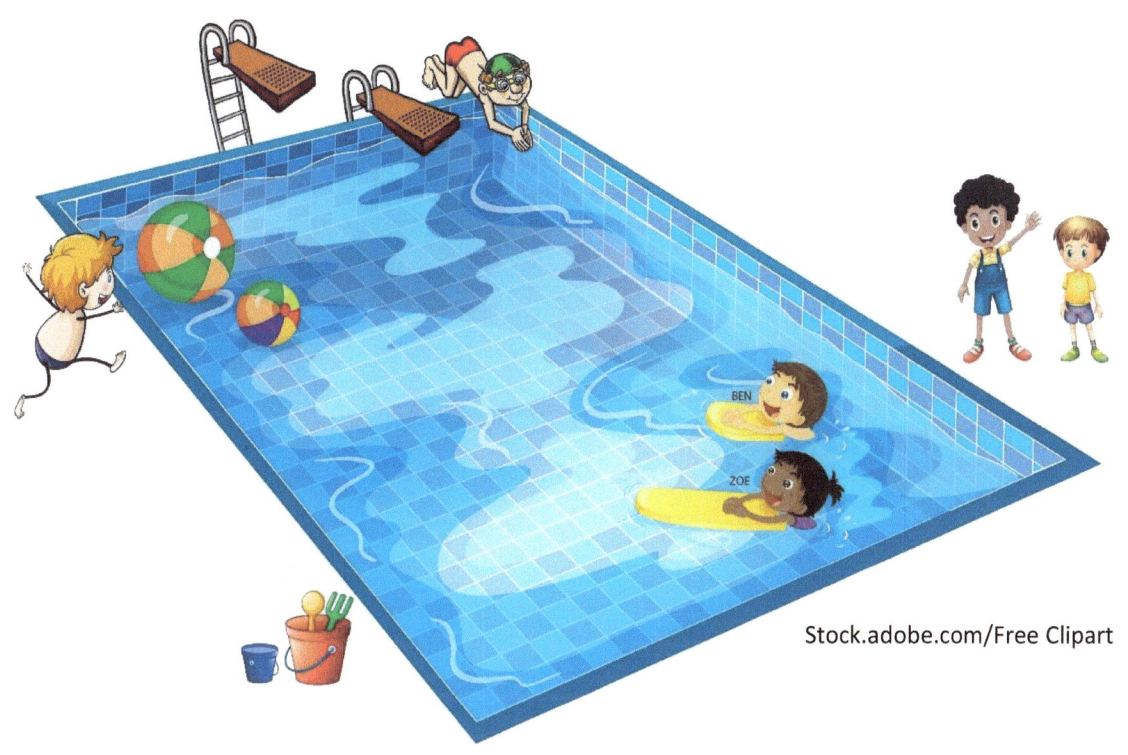

I wanna go to a restaurant
and to a public pool.
But with the COVID-19 monster around,
doing that is just not cool.

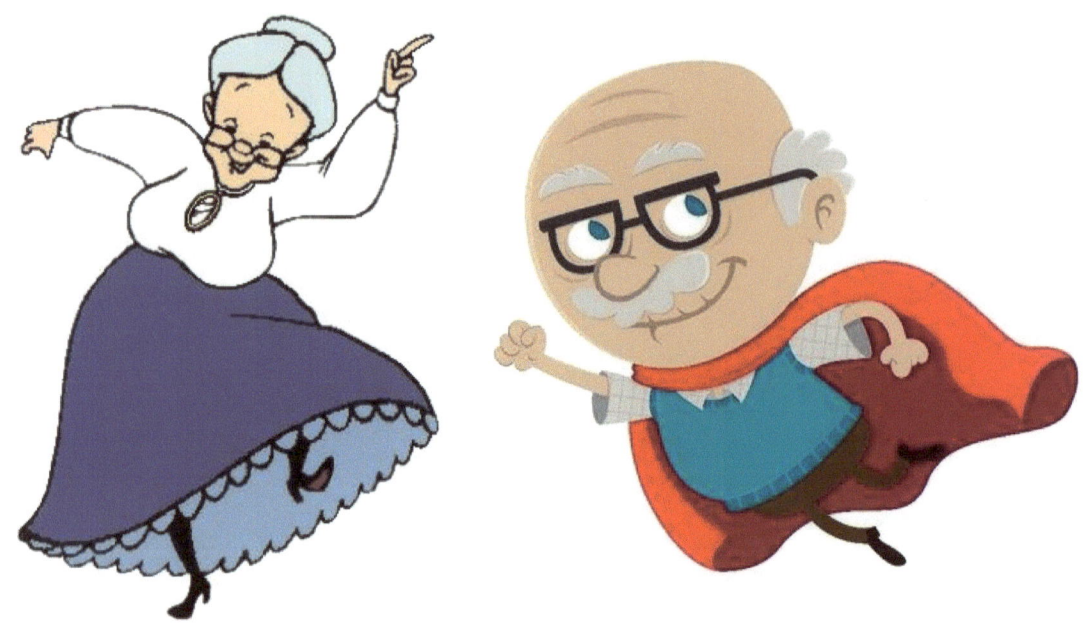

I wanna visit Mema and Dendaddy,

And play in the woods on the swing

But the COVID-19 monst**e**r could hop from me to them

and that wouldn't be a good thing.

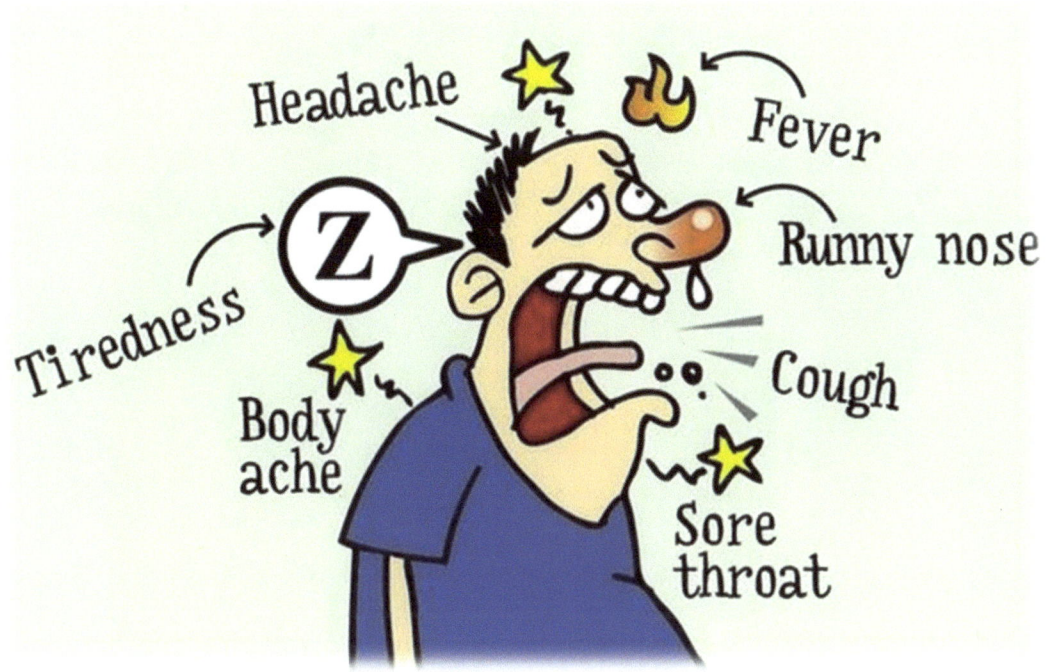

I don't wanna cause more COVID-19 deaths or terrible sickness in folks,

as the scientists and doctors search for the cure, and we wait with dreams and hopes.

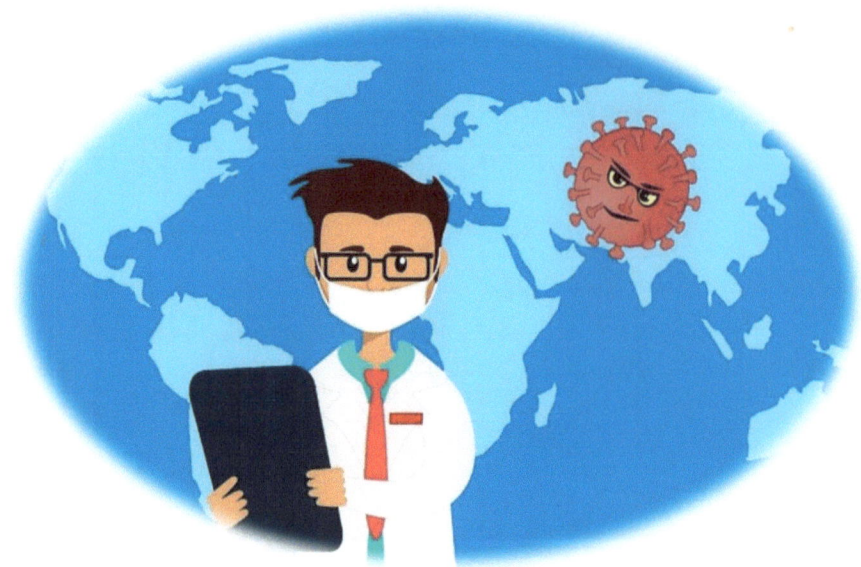

I don't wanna bring more danger to the brave caregivers who help,

But if I'm not careful, I could be one of the *asymptomatic*[2] killers myself.

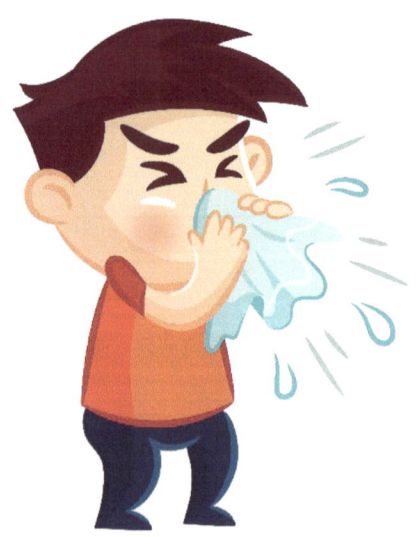

Elbow clipart cough, Transparent FREE, webstockreview.net

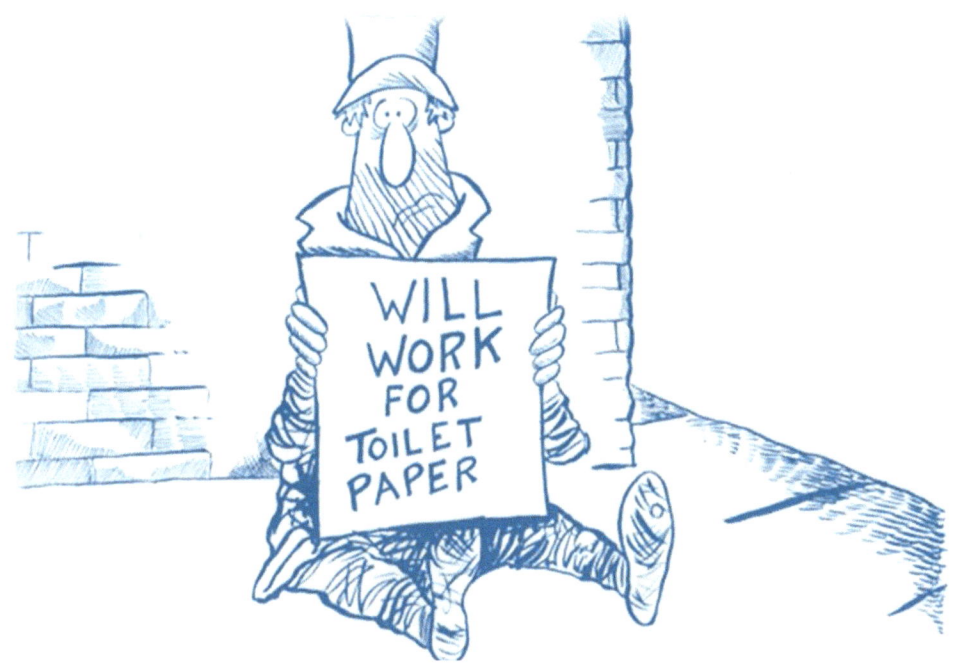

The Impact of COVID-19 in the Spring of 2020, RedState

So much hurt, anger, and pain is out there. So many are afraid.

I wanna help with all of it,

but I don't know how-- I'm dismayed.

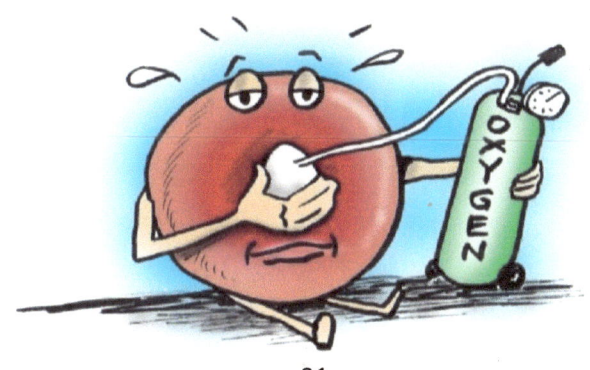

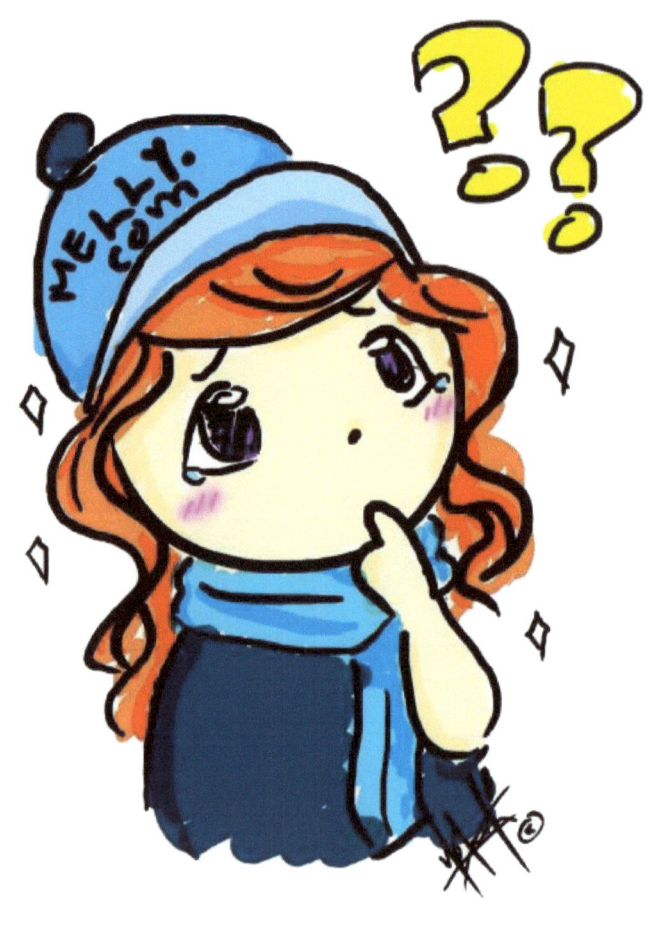

What can a person as young as I do?

In what ways can I step up?

Maybe I'll teach a couple of my friends about COVID-19.

Yeah, that's what's up!

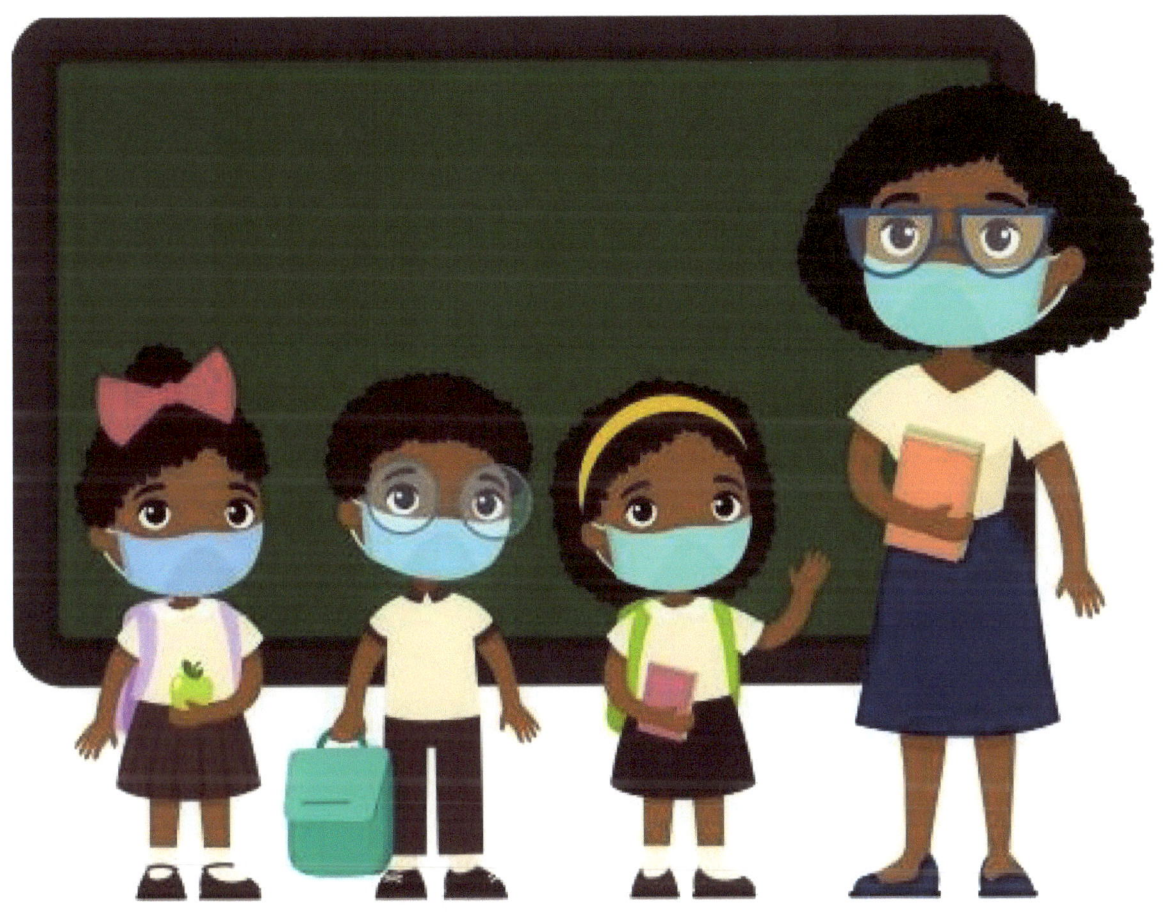

Pin on Kid Art, www.pinterest.com

I'll roll up my sleeves and help my mamma clean, clean, clean.
I'll wash my hands, front and back and all the places in-between.

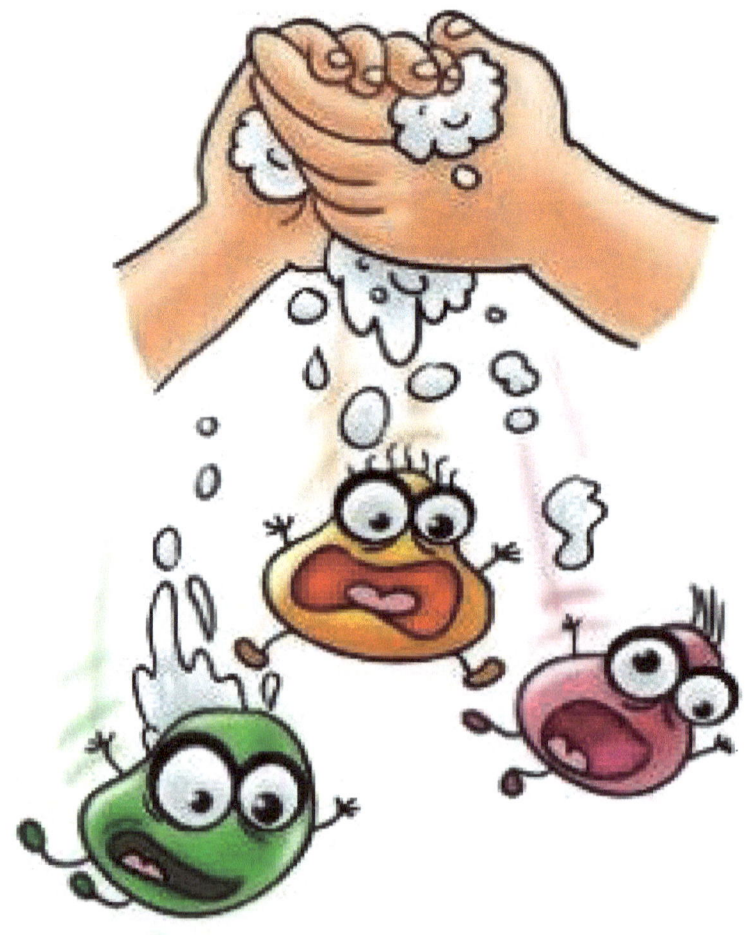

Longwood Elementary School, okaloosaschools.com

From what I hear, that's a **g**reat place to start with this COVID-19 monster thingy.

Soap and water, mas**k**s, and gloves are great weapons for this inv**i**sible enemy.

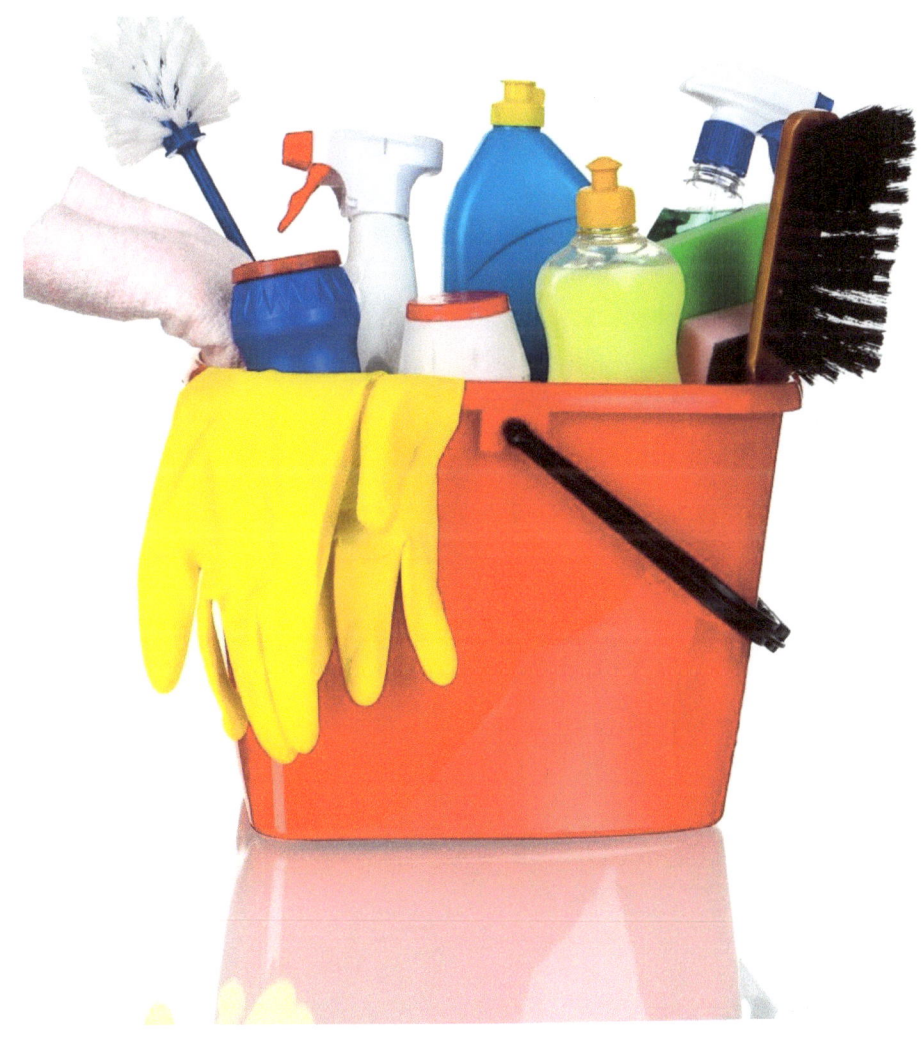

A**n**d I'll bake some cookies for my siblings

and save a few for myself.

I will wrap them up, like 3 or 4

and stack them on my be**d**room shelf.

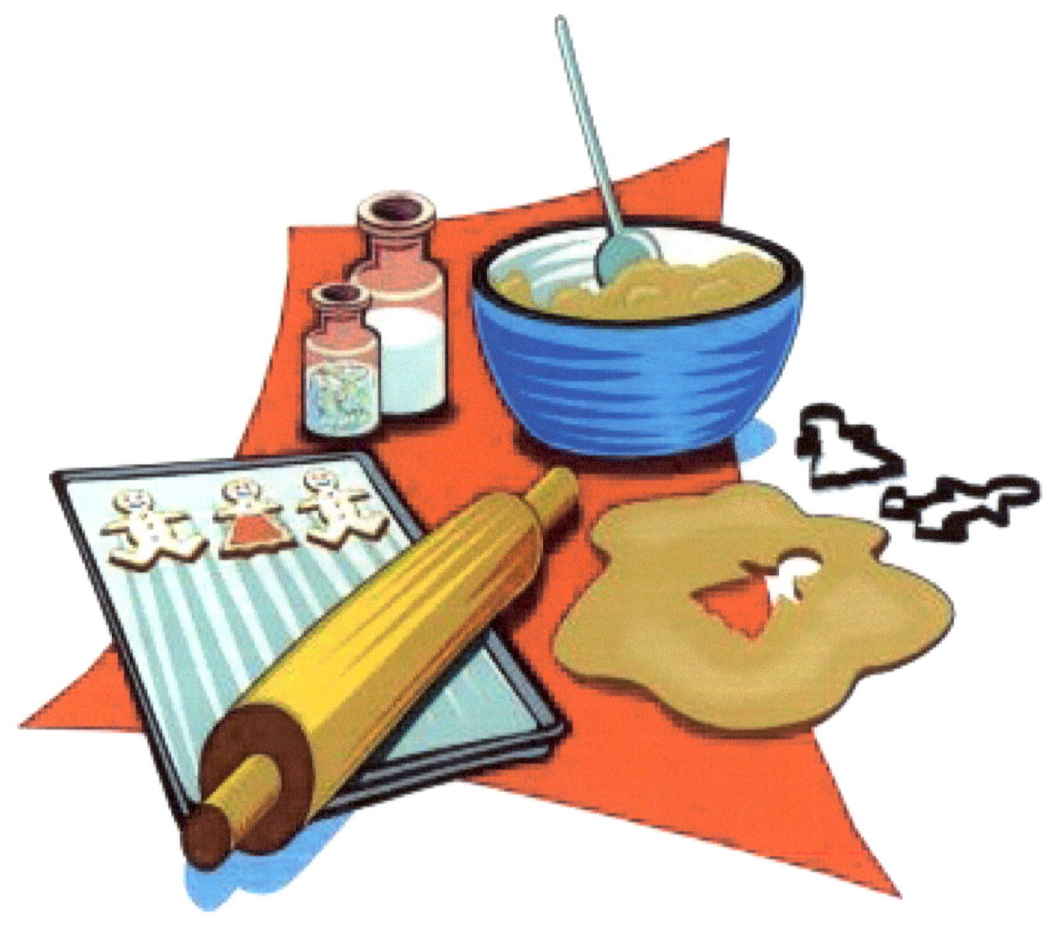

I will v**i**sit many place**s** through my **c**ollection of books and in my imaginati**o**n.

I wil**l** travel t**o** other lands and times, fa**r** away, and continue my education.

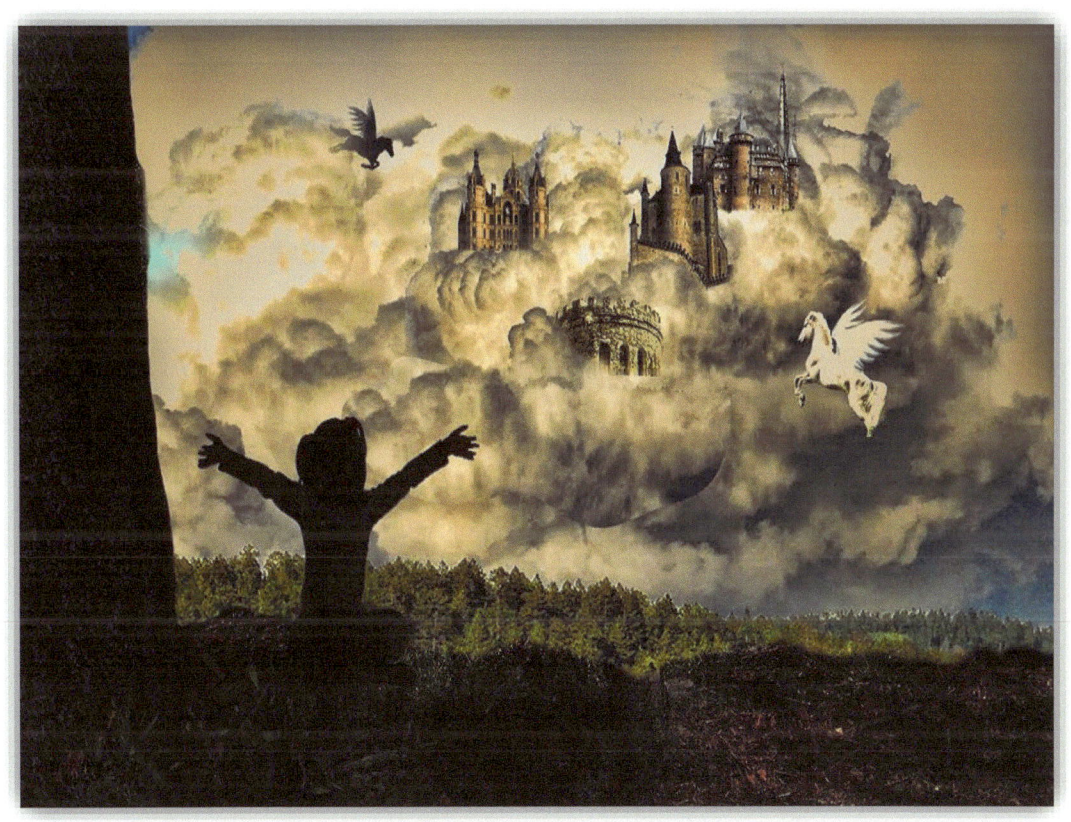

I don't w**a**nna spread COVID-19 mons**t**ers in swimming pools where others m**i**ght get sick.

We already can't go to **o**ur schools right now. Somethings gotta change --- and quick!

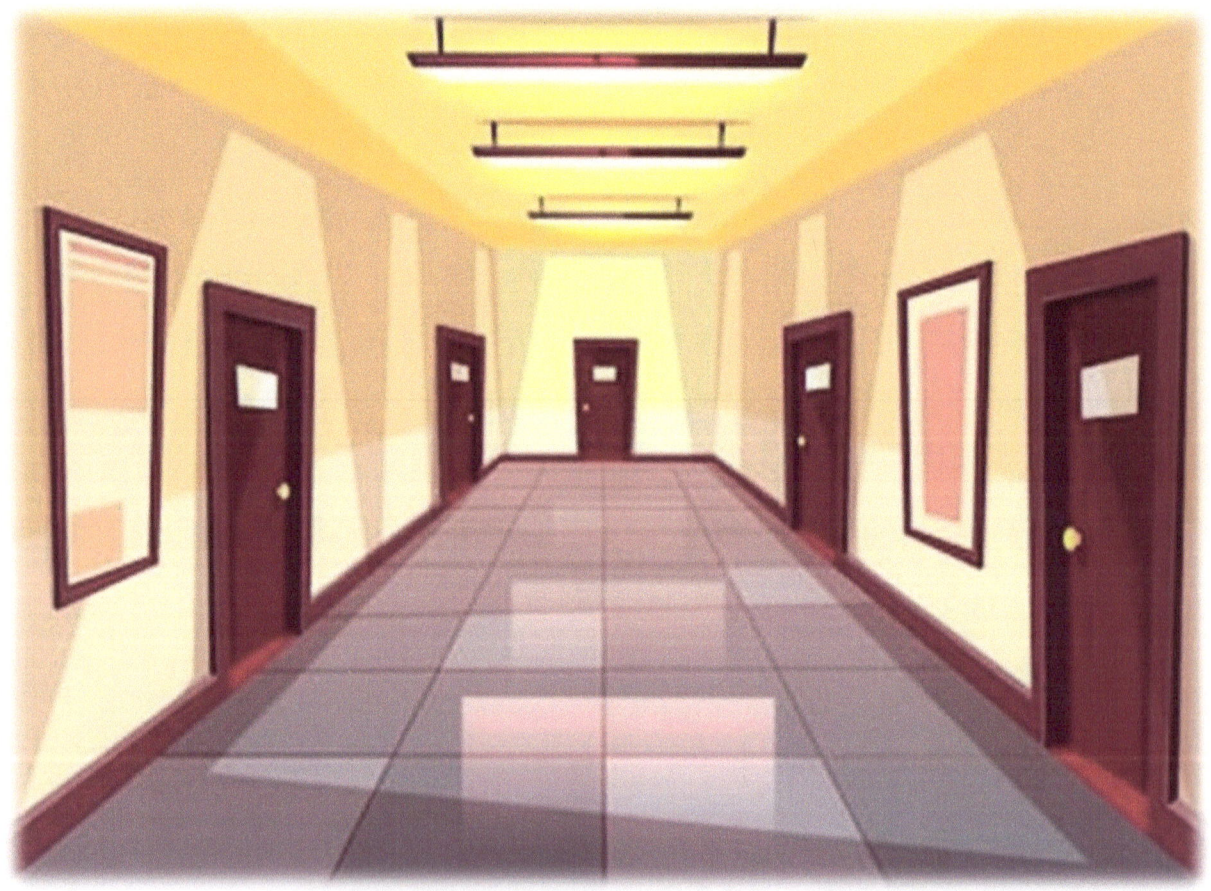

Hallway Images, Stock Photos & Vectors, Shutterstock

So I'll just have a splash party

in my yard with the sprinkler on the grass.

I will even pretend I'm fishing,

and catch lots of sea bass.

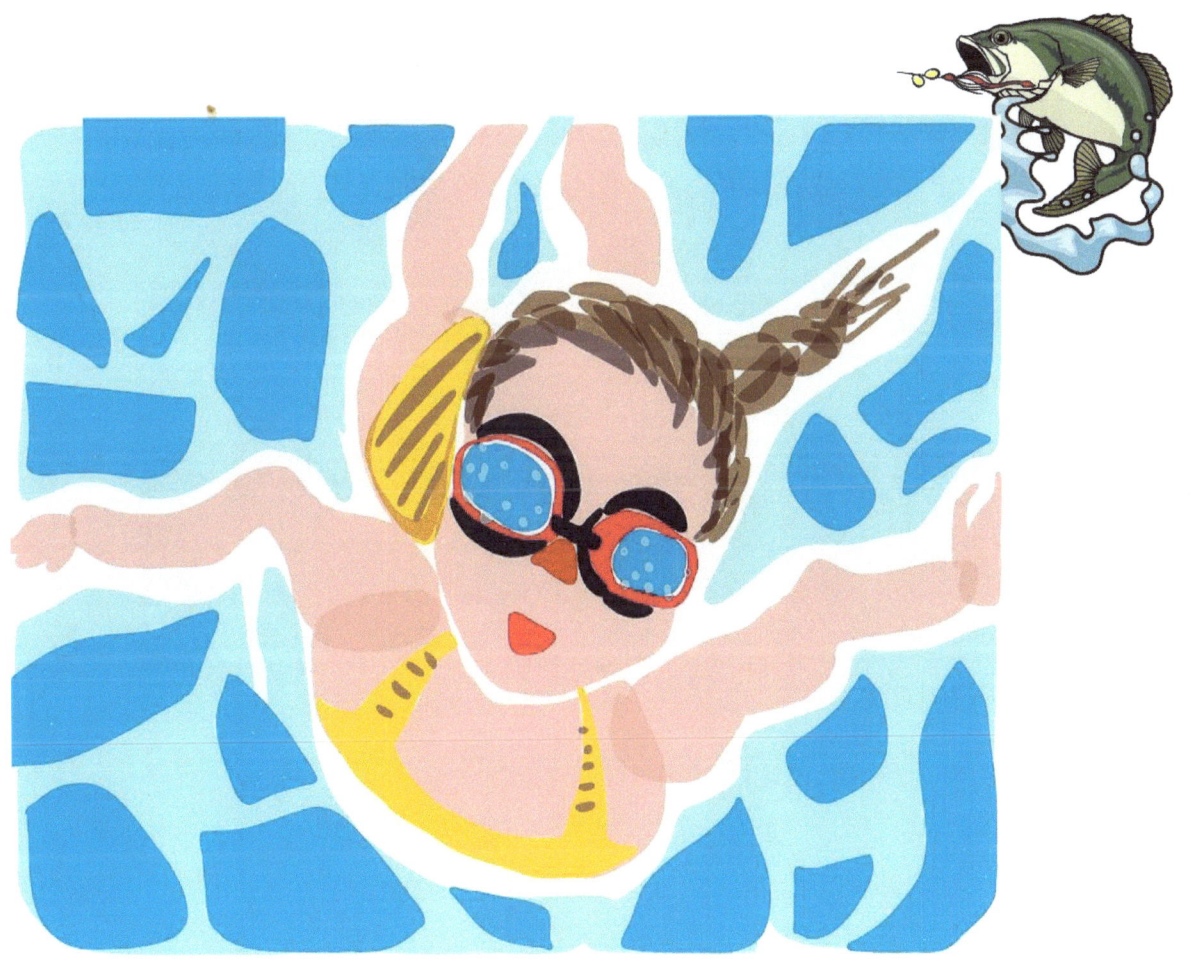

I will use my artwo*r*k

to make c*a*rds for the sick and elderly.

And deliver them on my bicycle

to their porches, happily.

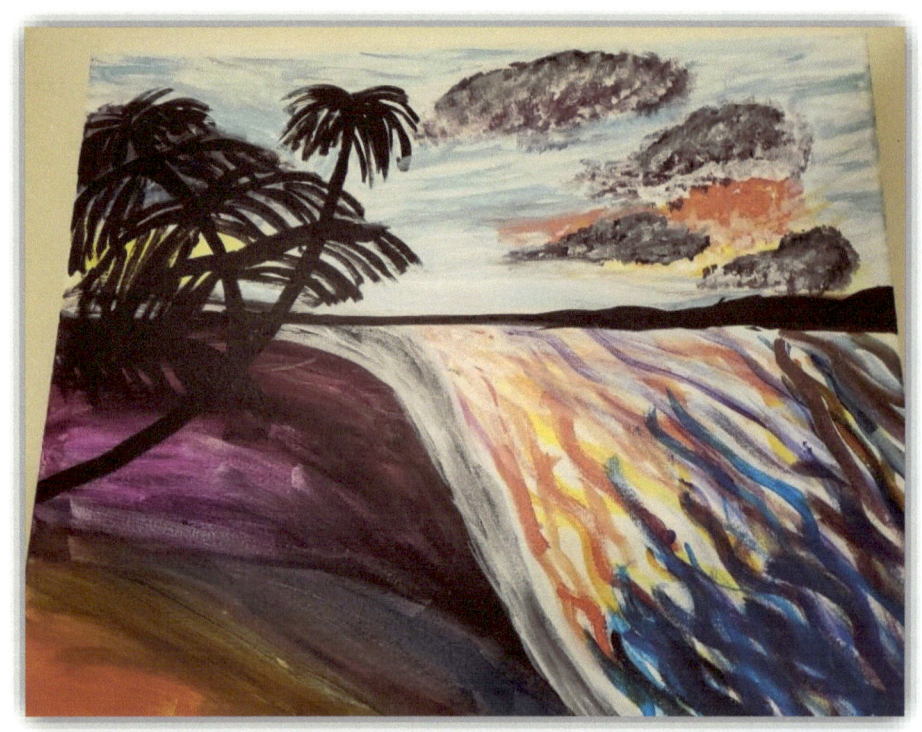

Painted by Niyah Mason (age 11)

{Instructor: Muse Paint Bar}

While I miss my Meema and Dendaddy, and can't ride my bike to their place. I'll ask my mom and dad to Facetime them, to see their smiling faces.

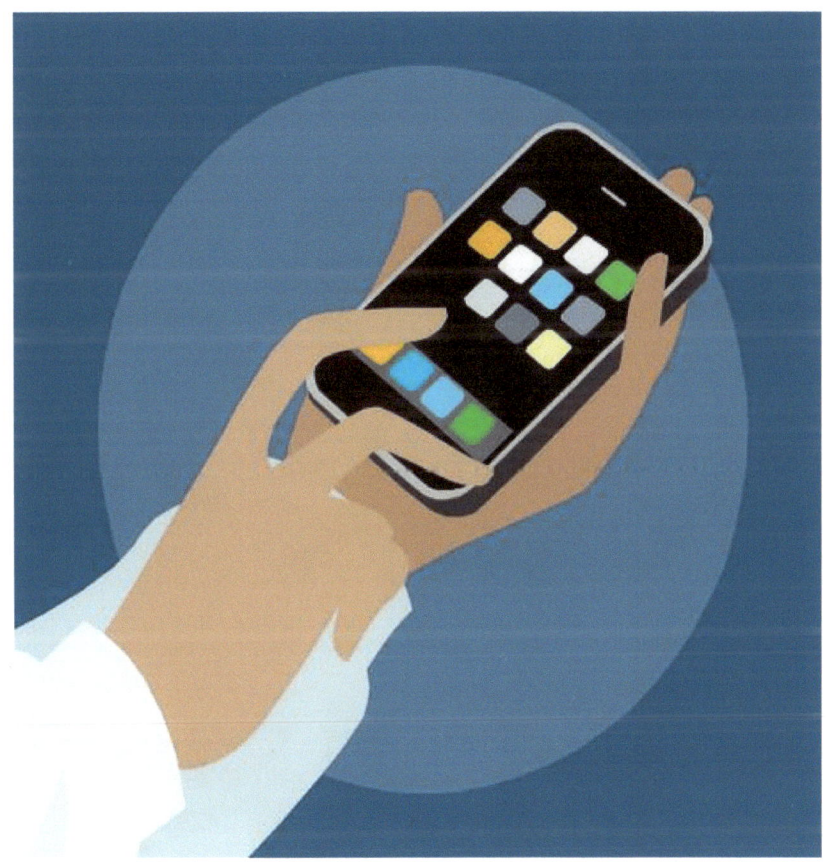

The COVID-19 monster said that we should be afraid.

It's hard to have hope at all.

But Meema and Dendaddy told us once,

"When we know Jesus,

we are greater than them all."

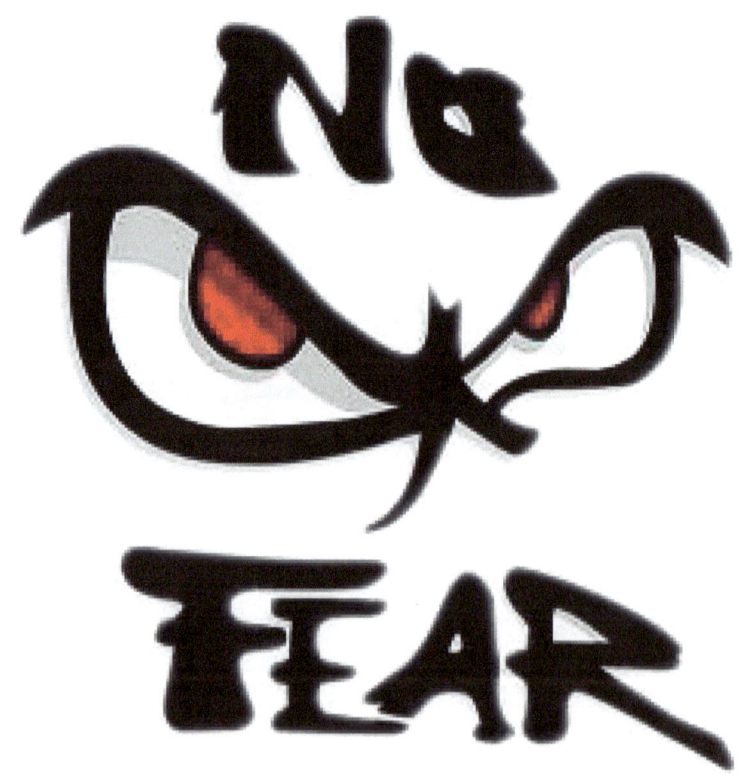

PART 3
Tellin' It Like Some Perceive It to Be

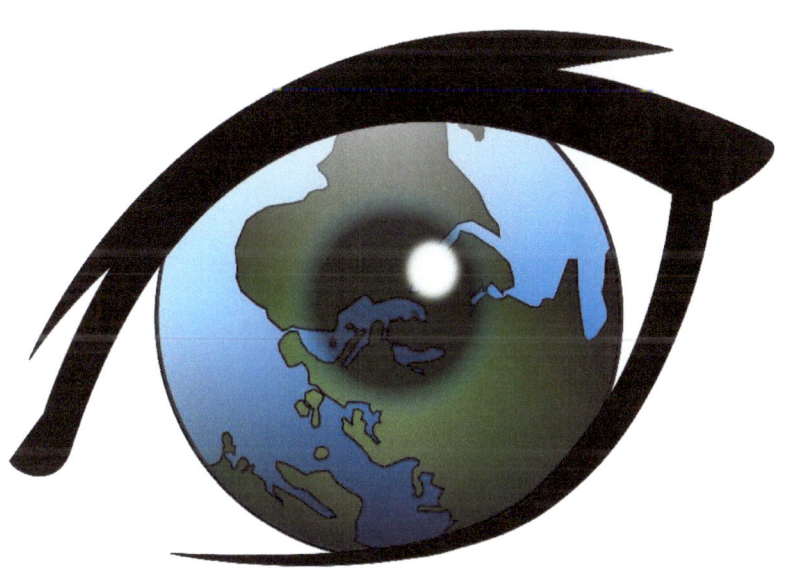

Affection During This Time of COVID-19

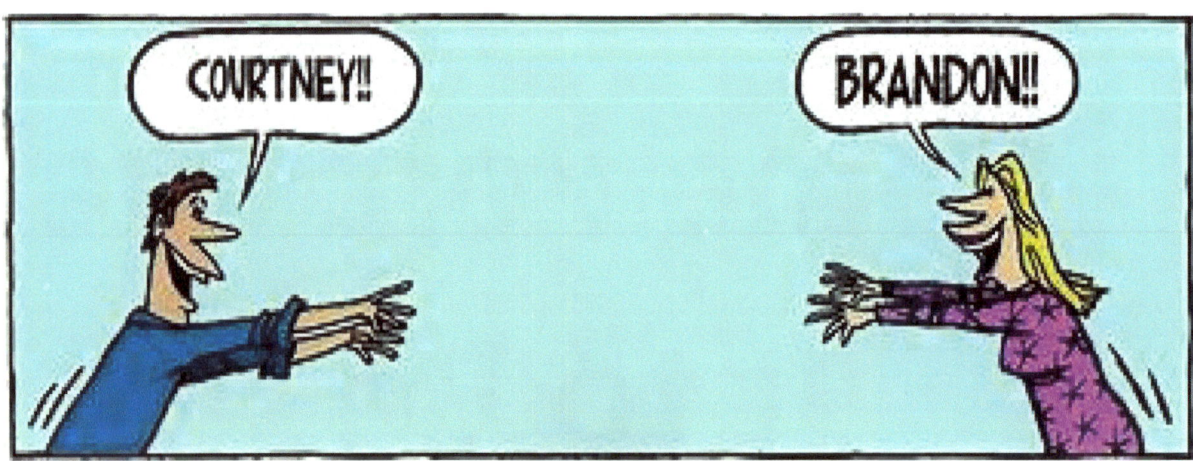

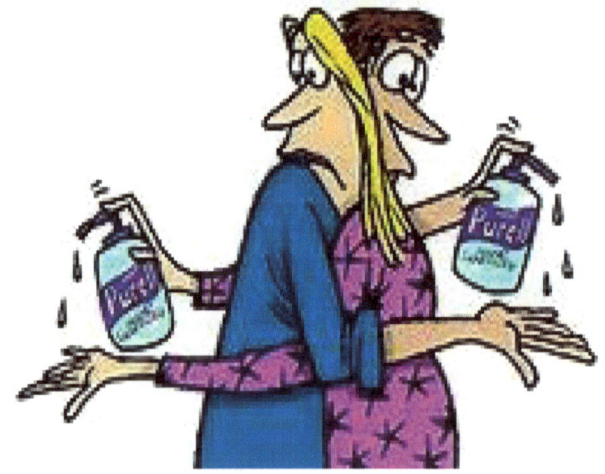

Editorial Cartoon: Courtney and Brandon-opinion-Austin, Austin American-Stateman

Religion During This Time of COVID-19

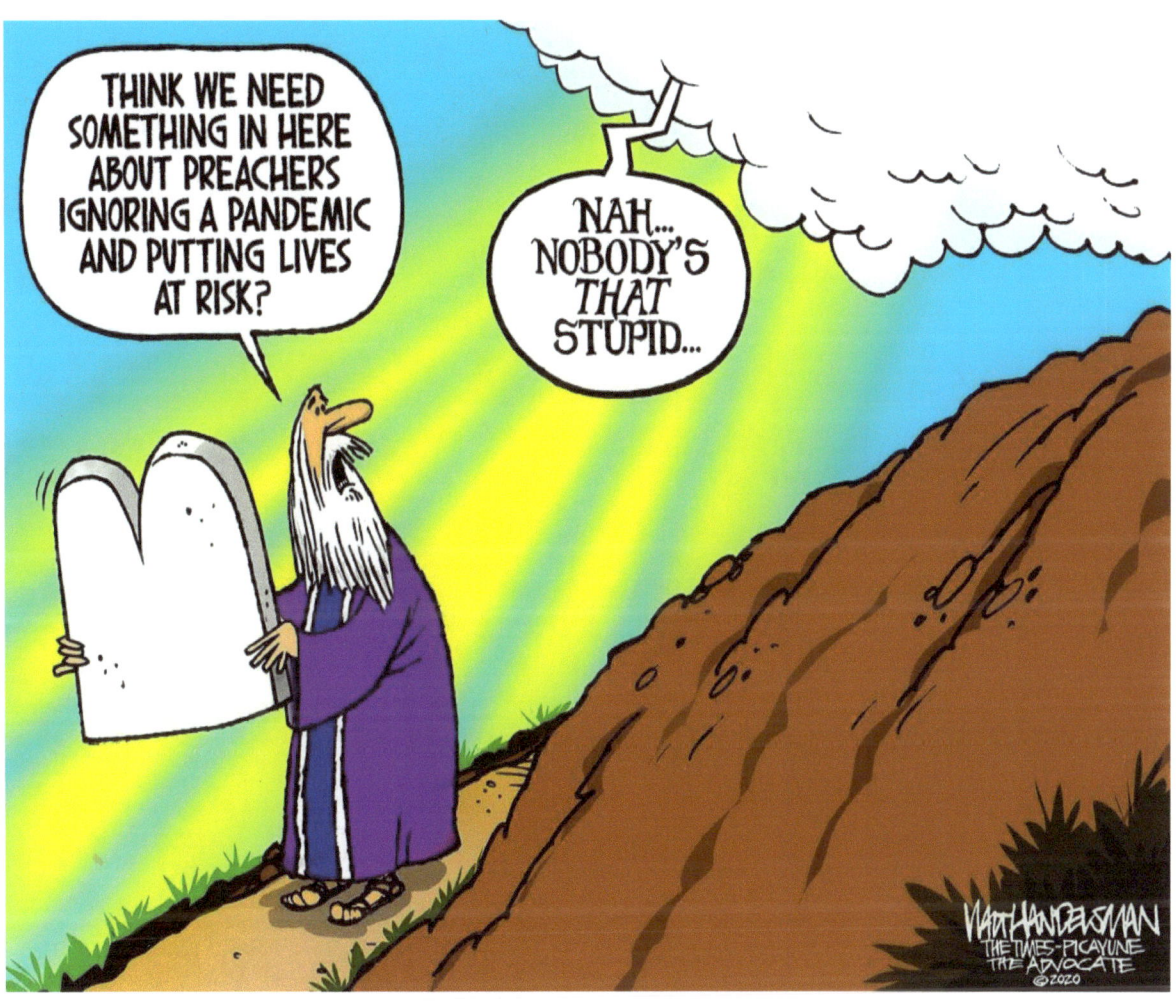

Protected Commodities During This Time of COVID-19

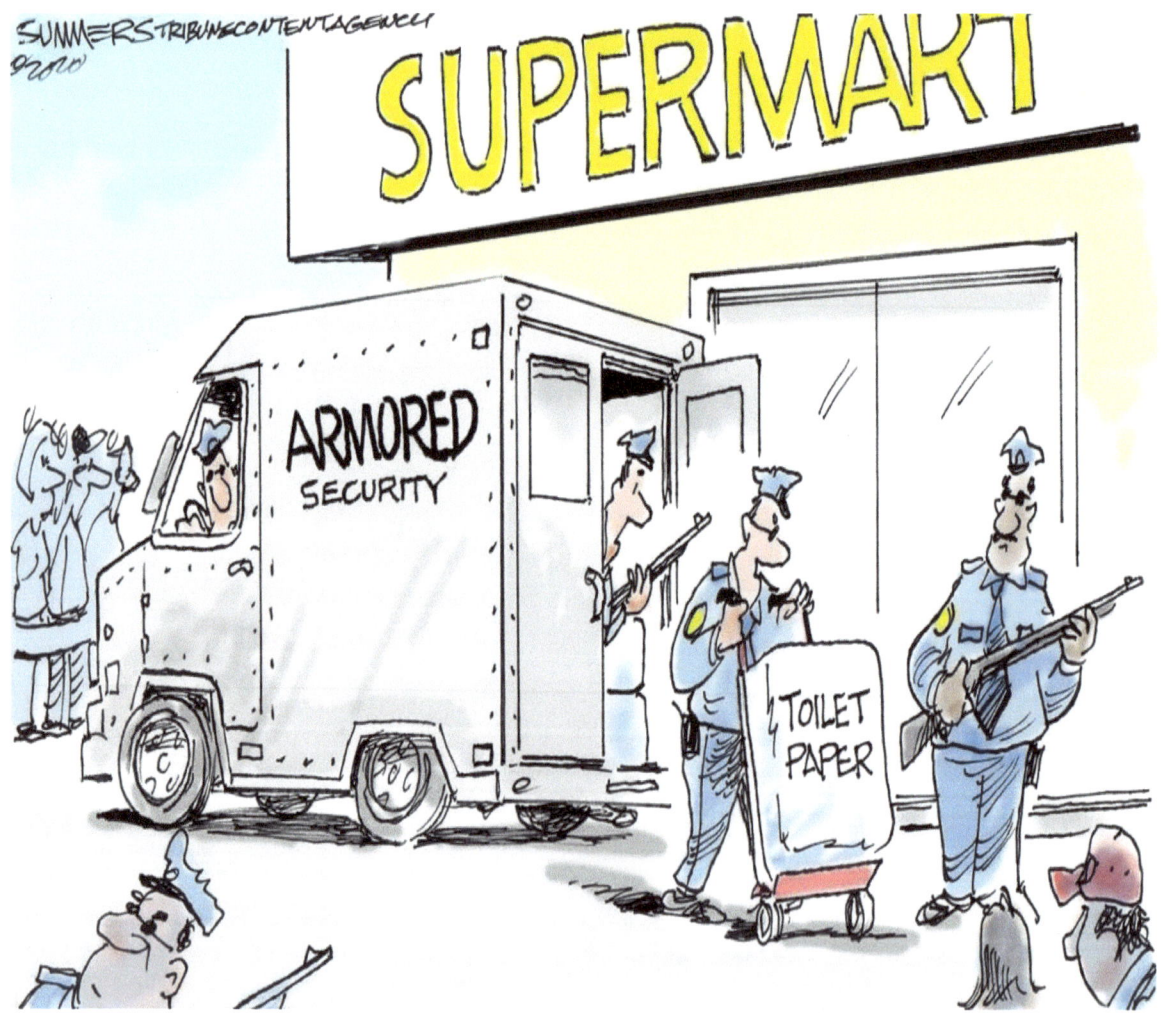

Republicans, Democrats and the Coronavirus: U.S. News and World Reports

Shopping During This Time of COVID-19

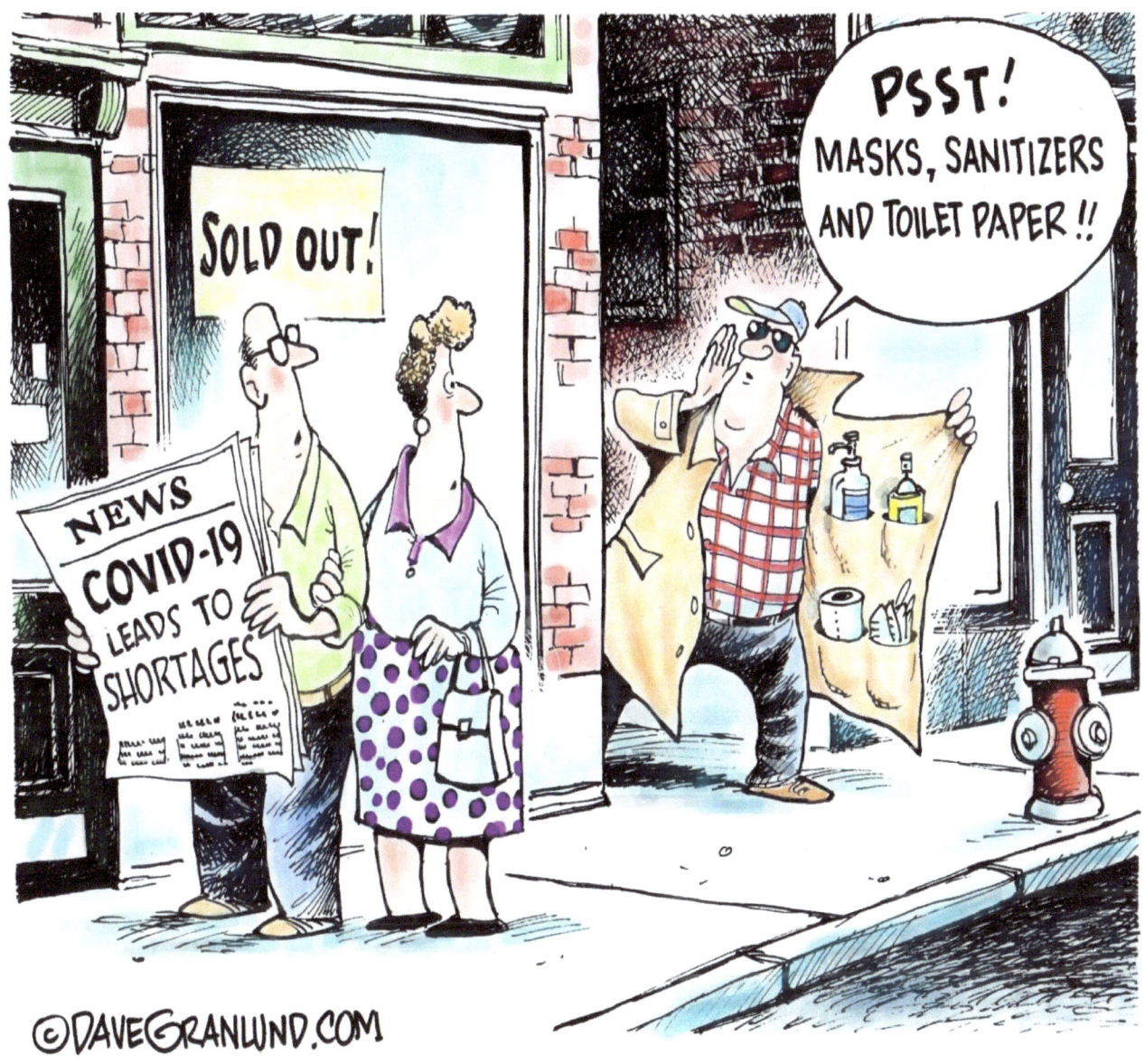

Granlund Cartoon: Staying Safe-Opinion-Erie Times-News, GoErie.com

Quarantining During This Time of COVID-19

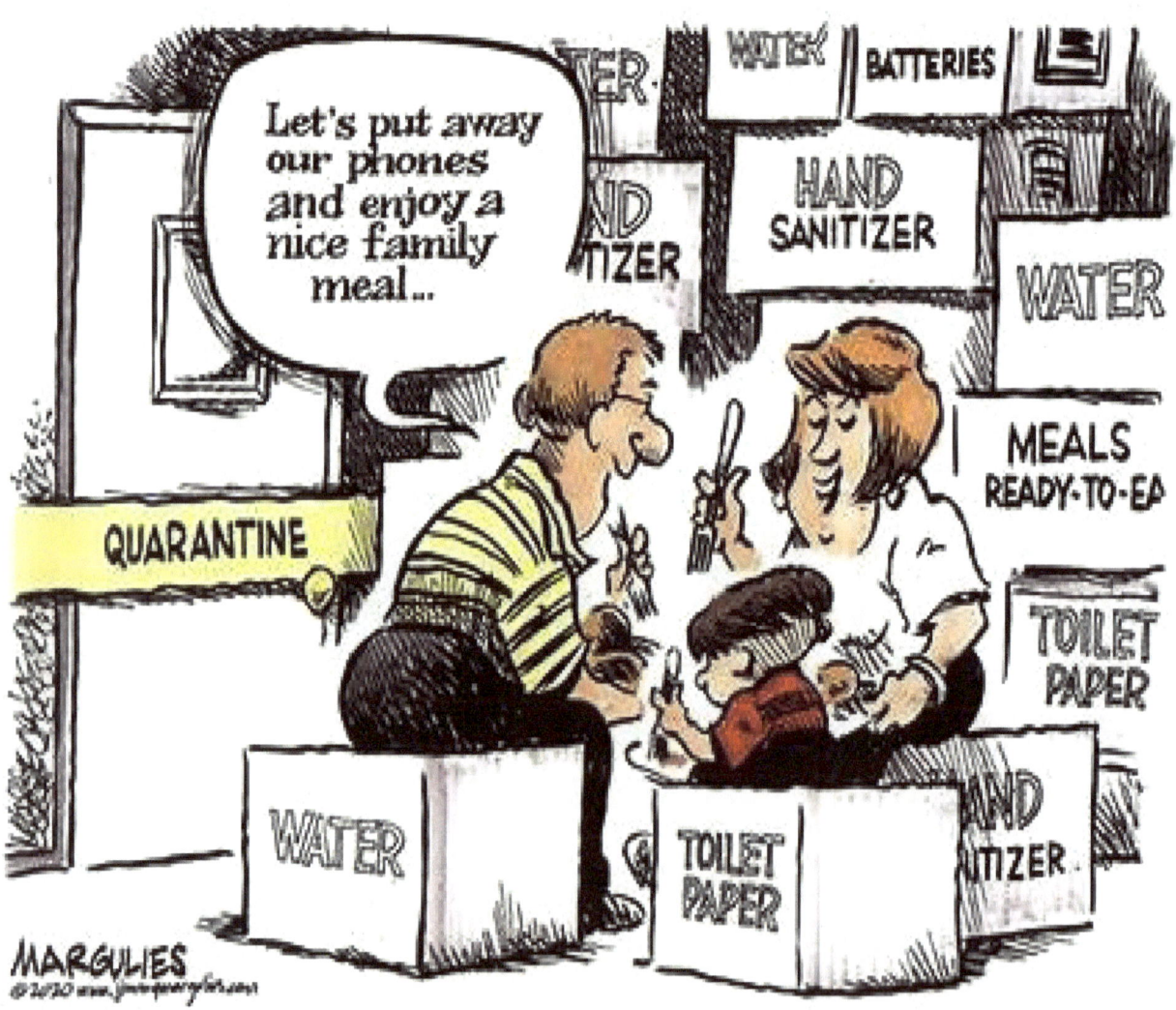

Coronavirus Quarantine, Cage Post

Fake News and Hypocrisy During This Time of COVID-19

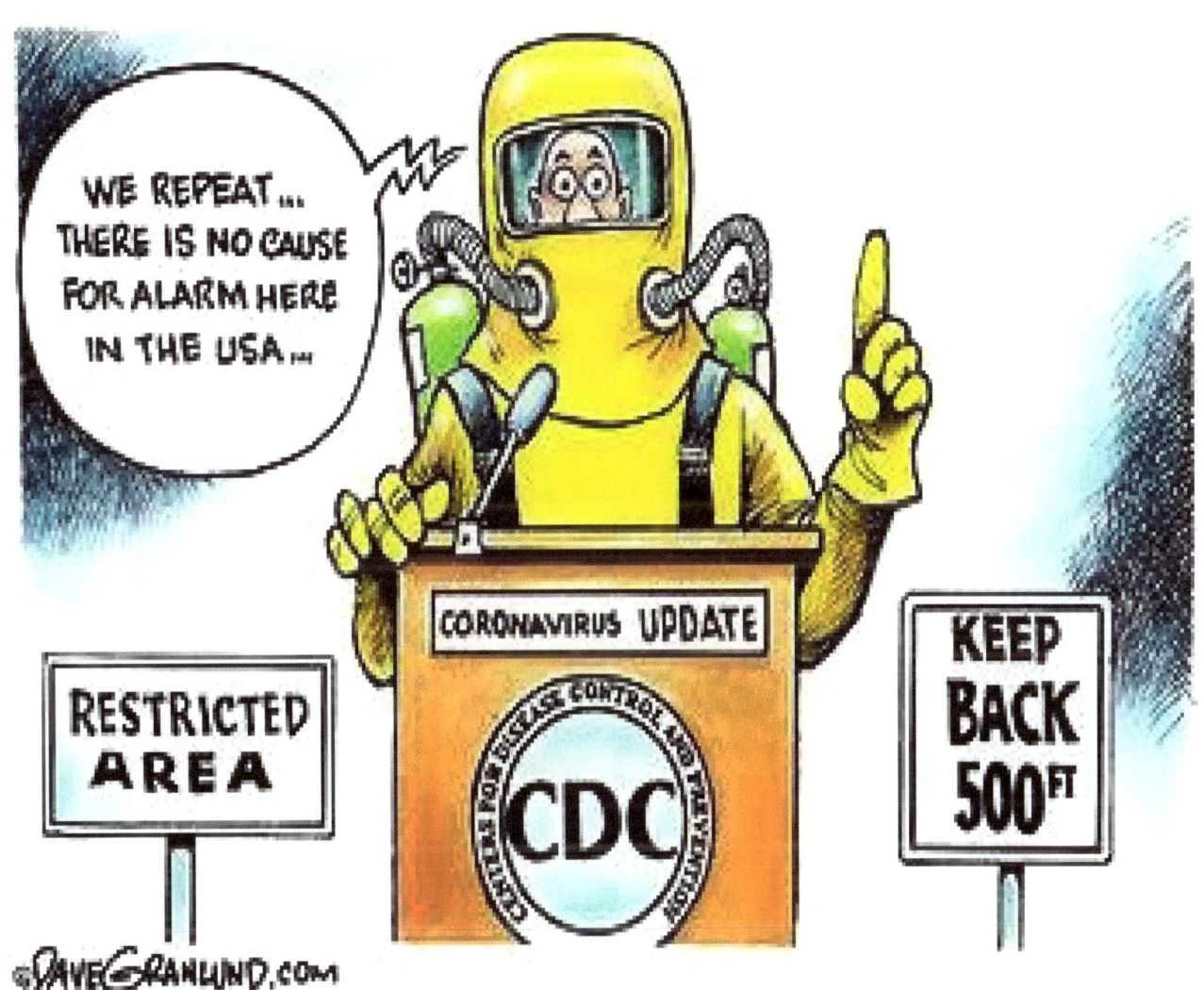

Dave Granlund-Editorial Cartoons and Illustrations, Davegranlund.com

Testing During This Time of COVID-19

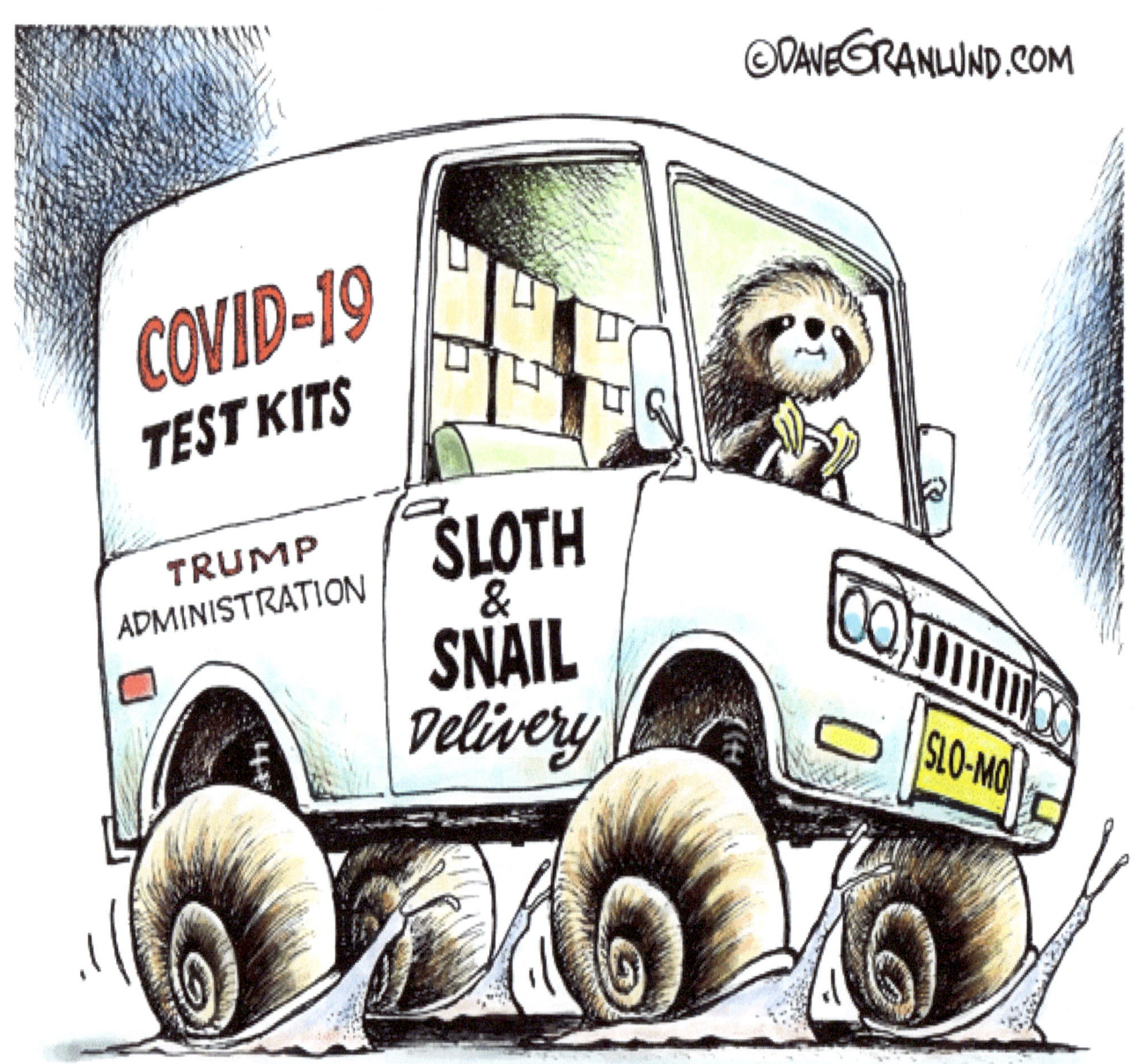

Granlund Cartoons: COVID-19 Test Kits-opinion-fosters, Foster's Daily Democrat

Mixed Messaging During This Time of COVID-19

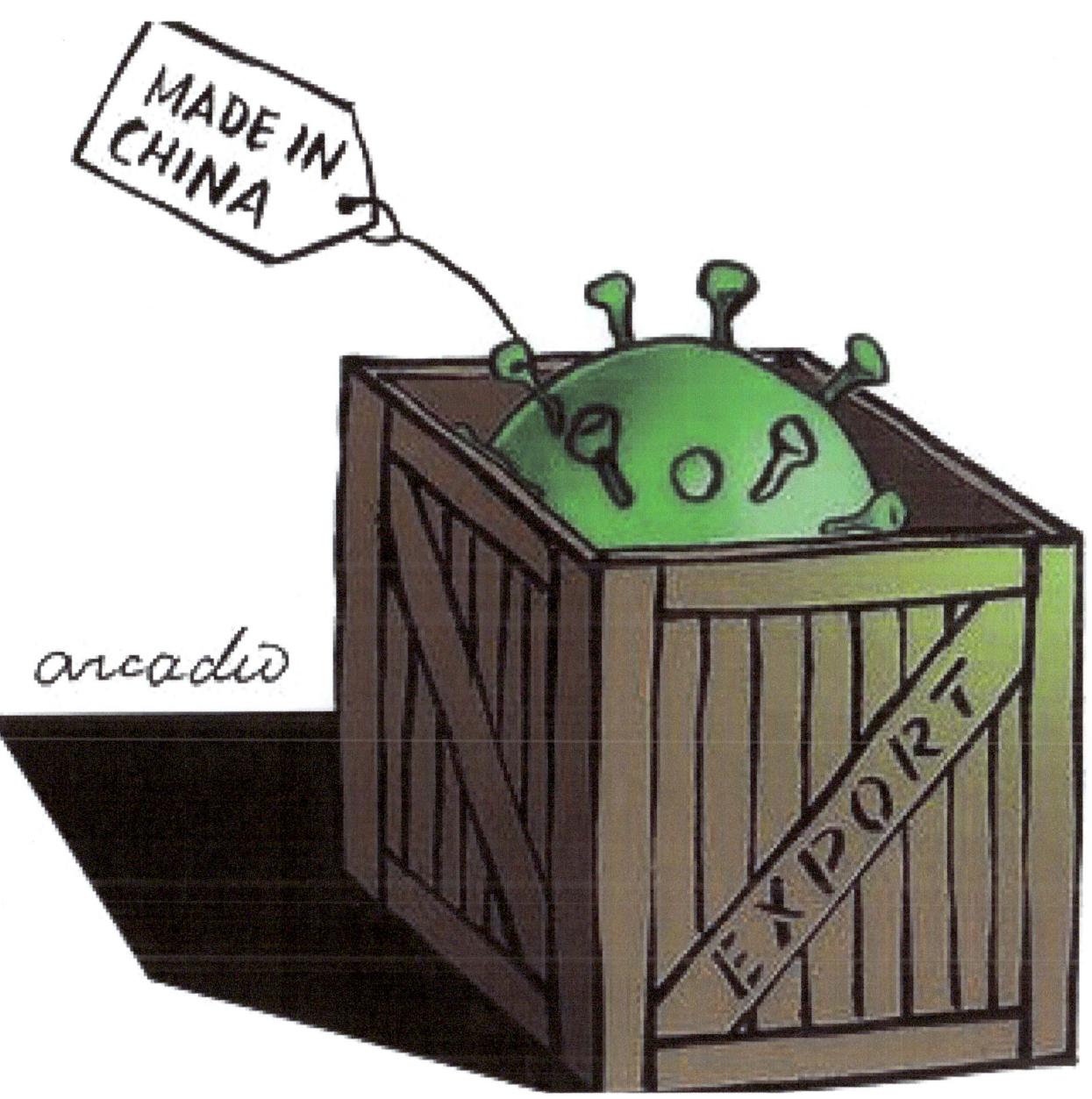

Guest View: Get the facts on the Coronavirus, COVID-19, Billings Gazette

Political Propaganda During This Time of COVID-19

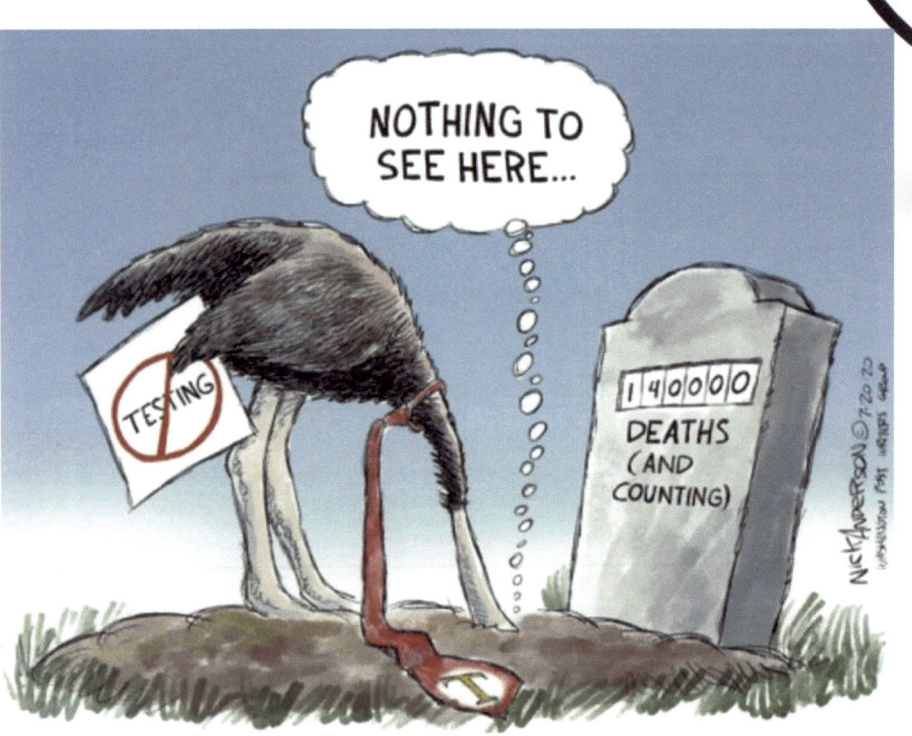

Nick Anderson Copyright 2020,
Andrews McMeel Syndication

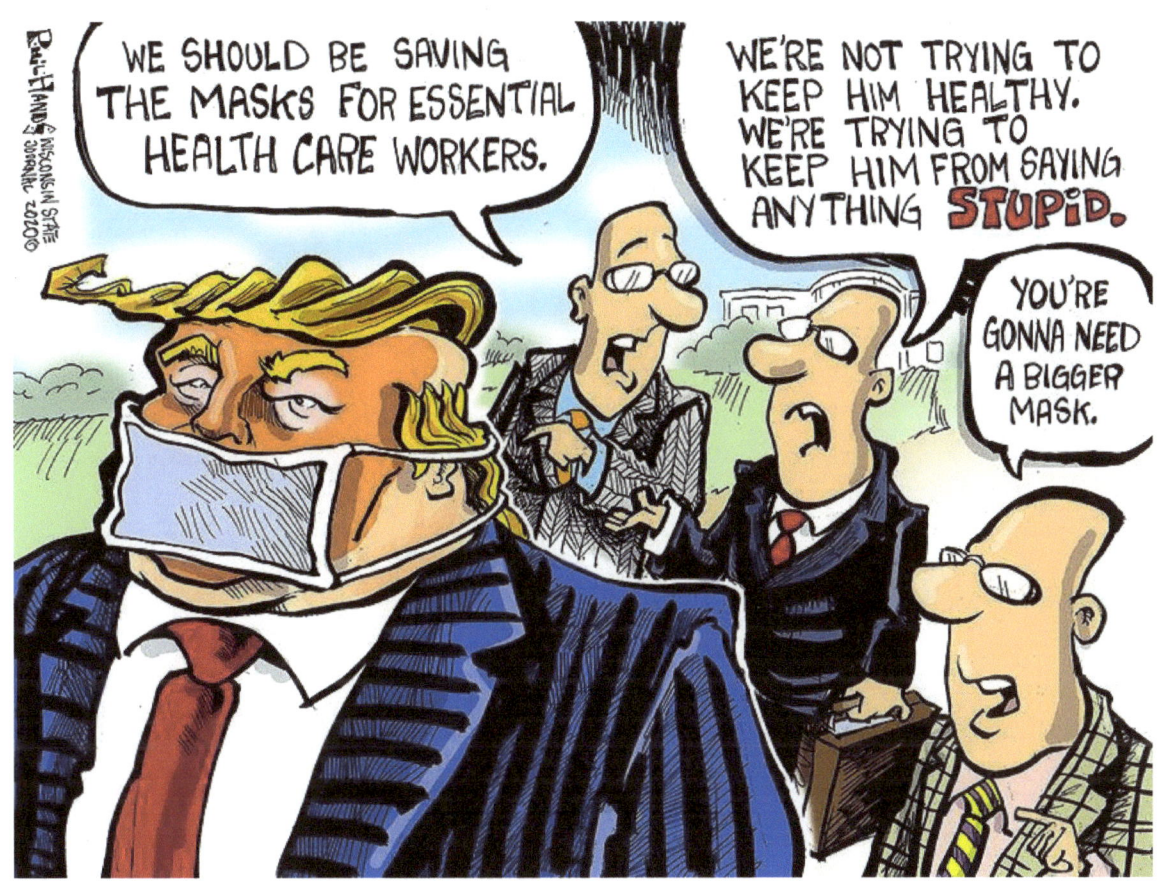

Hands on Wisconsin: Trump will need a bigger Coronavirus

More Propaganda Advertising During This Time of COVID-19

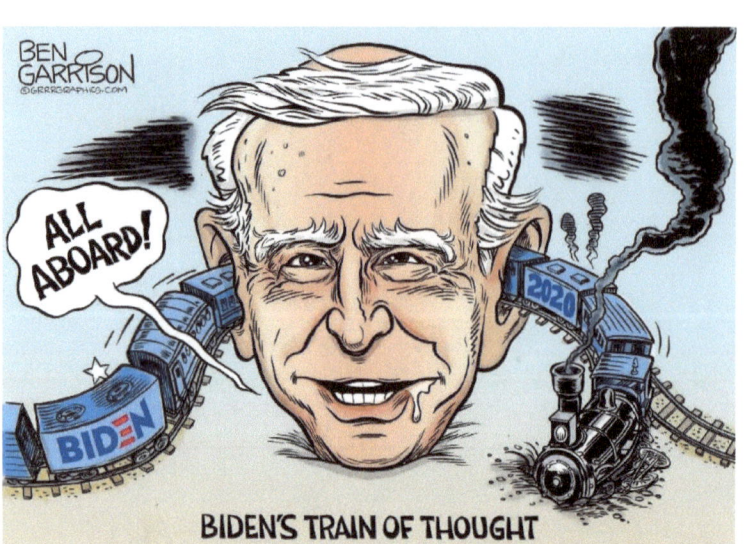

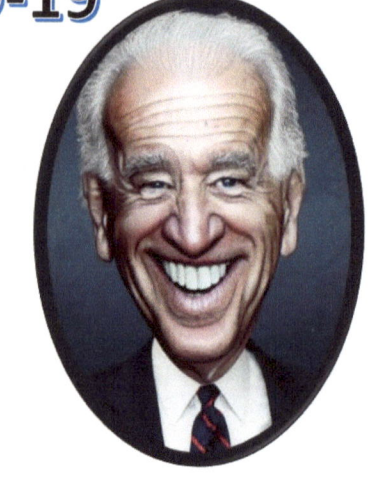

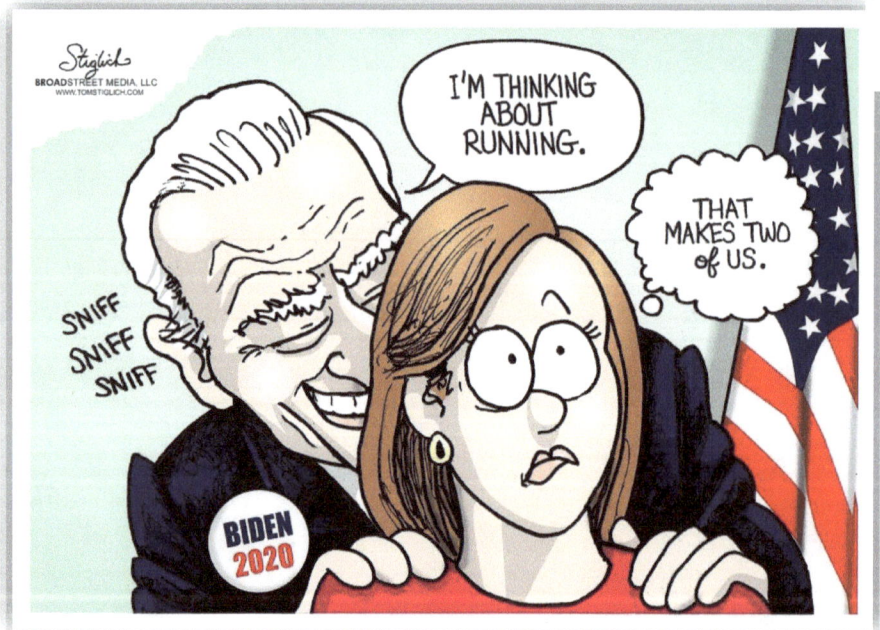

Ben Garrison Cartoon, Conservativedailynews.com

The guillotine of public opinion
Comes for Joe Biden, Personal Liberty

Misguided Youth Thinking During This Time of COVID-19

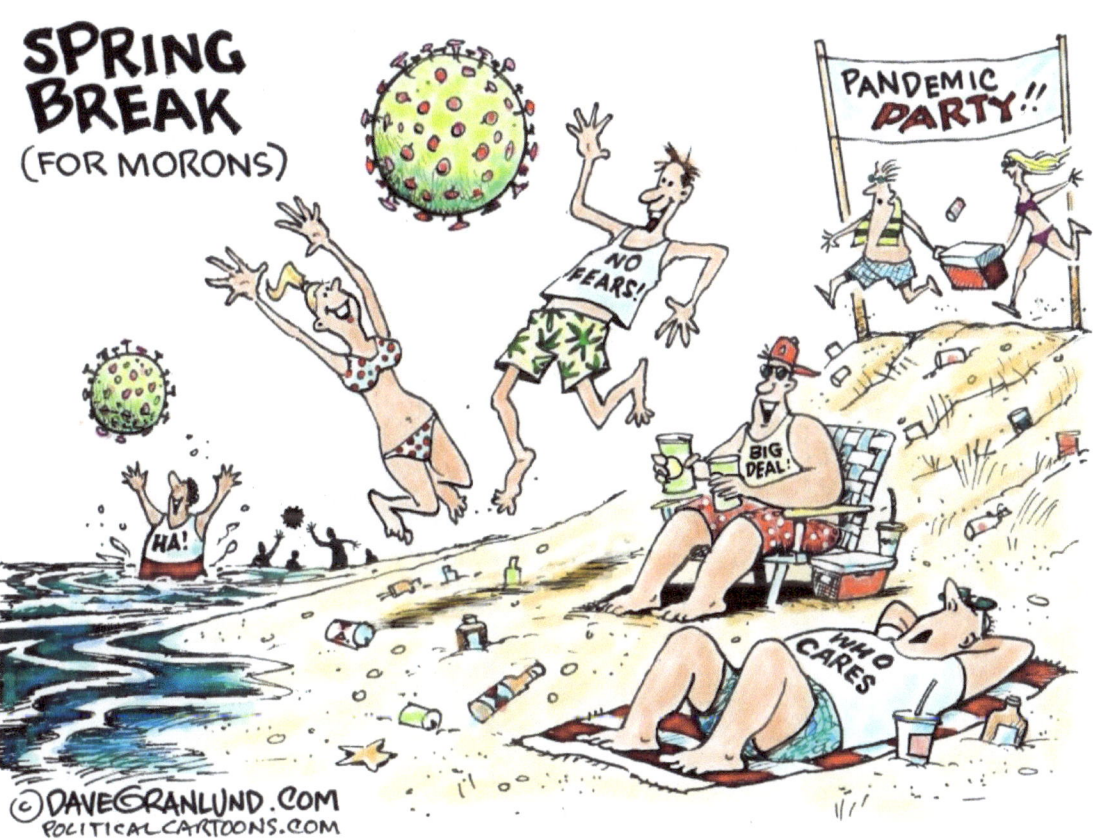

DaveGranlund.com, Political Cartoons.com, Times News

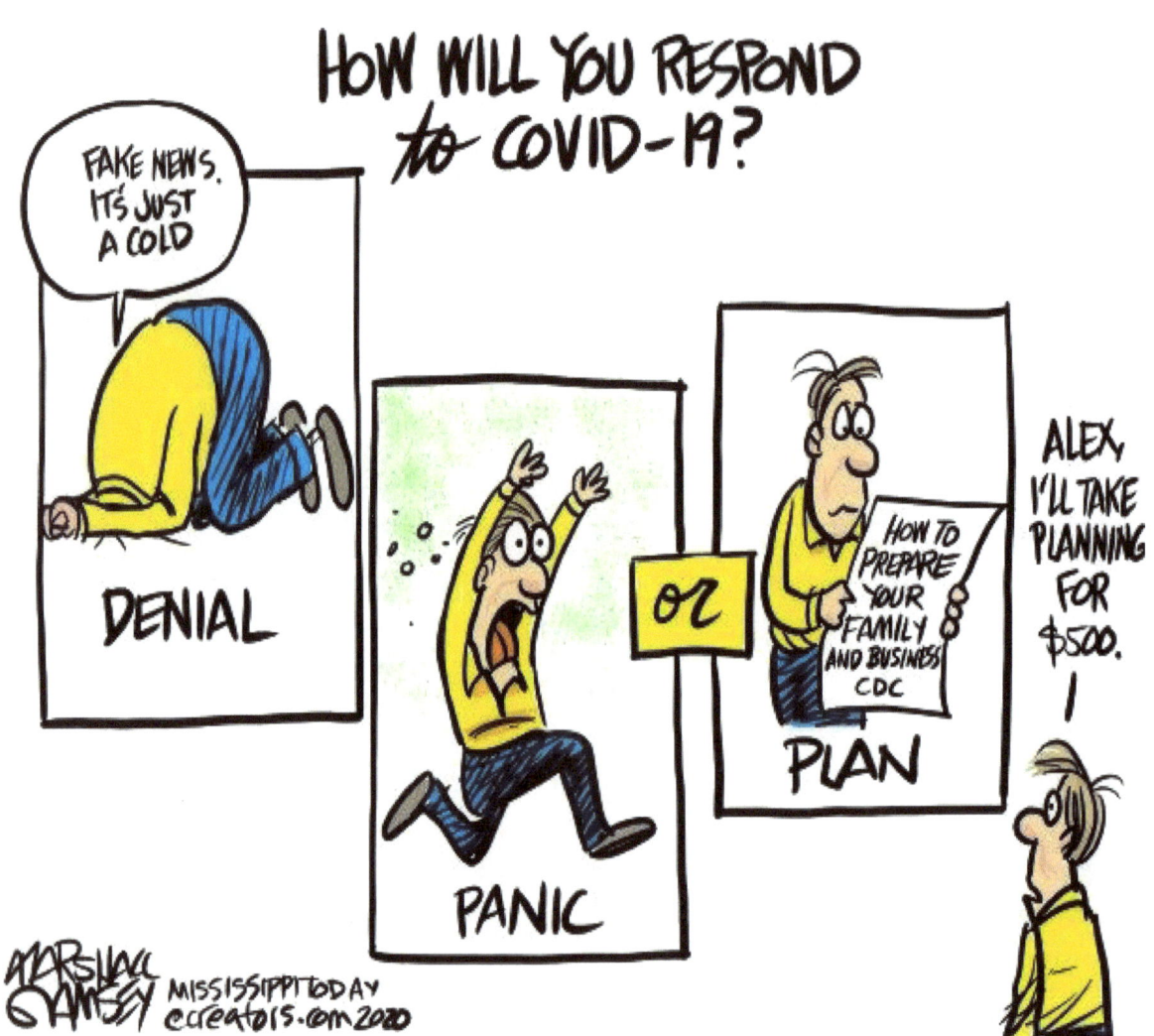

Marshall Gamsey, Mississippi Today, Creators.com 2020

NEVER FORGET our Heroes

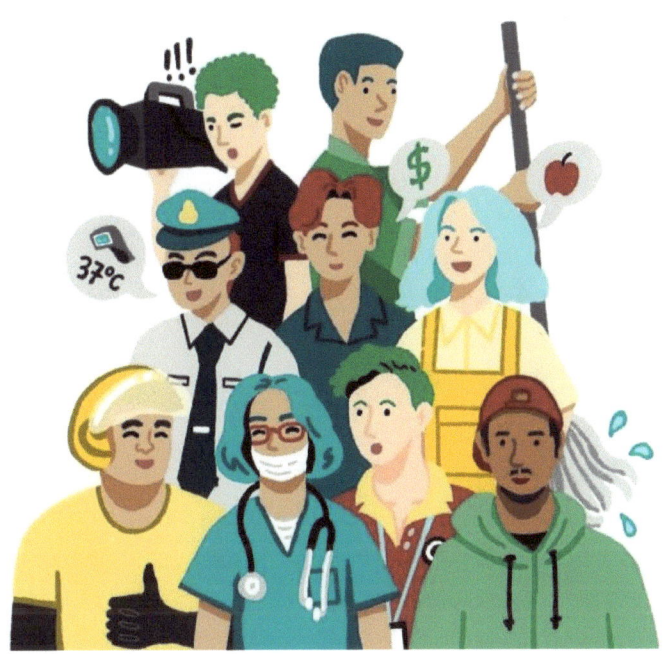

NEVER FORGET: The Unsung Heroes of Today's Battle Against... Wheninmanila.com

Health Care Workers	Retailers	Scientists
Refuse Collectors	Custodians	Grocery Store Workers
Fast Food Workers	First Responders	Police Officers
Postal Workers	Delivery Workers	Factory Workers
Child Care Workers	Teaching Staff	Government Workers
Drug Store Workers	Nursing Home Staff	Congress Workers
Fire Fighters	US Armed Forces	Bankers

Citizens who listen to scientist and doctors by wearing mask/shields and practice social distancing during this time of COVID-19

News media that reports FACTS and the TRUTH

Active volunteers, unselfish givers & so many unknown others

WE THANK YOU!

Preventing the Spread of COVID-19

COVID-19 has also been proven to spread back and forth between animals (such as pets) and humans.

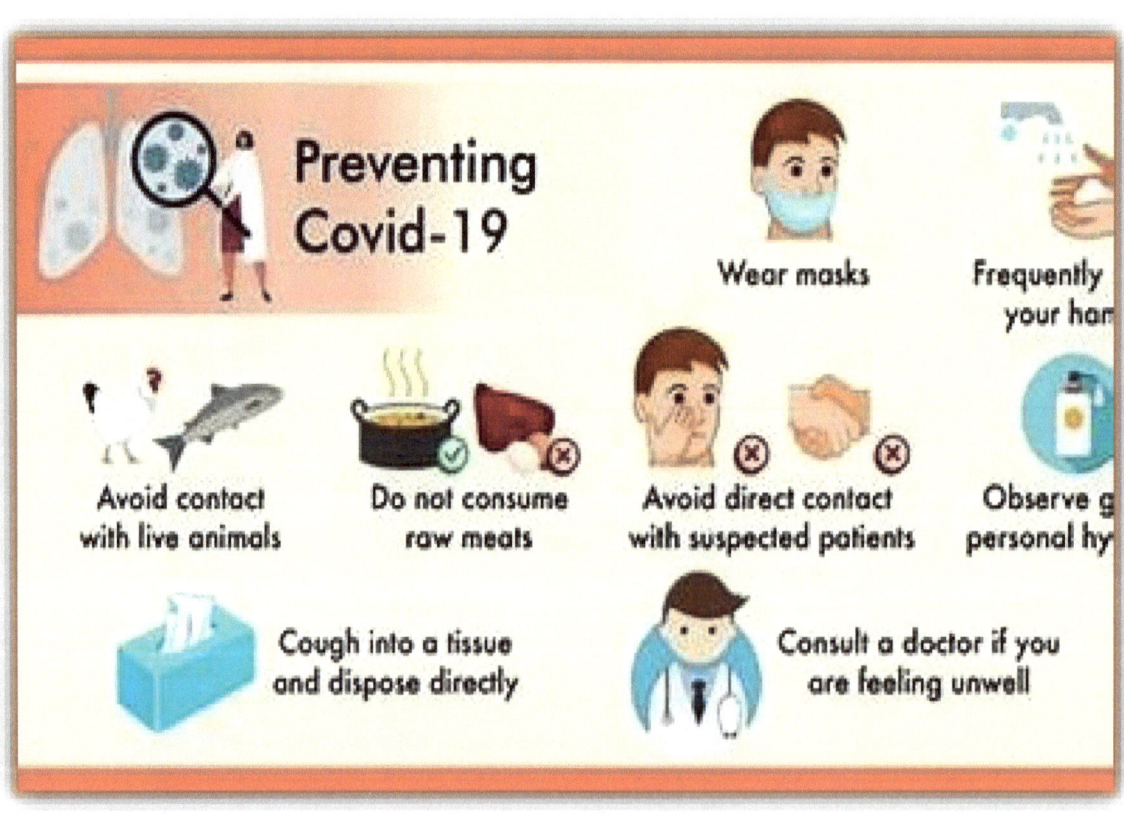

WHAT ABOUT MY PETS?

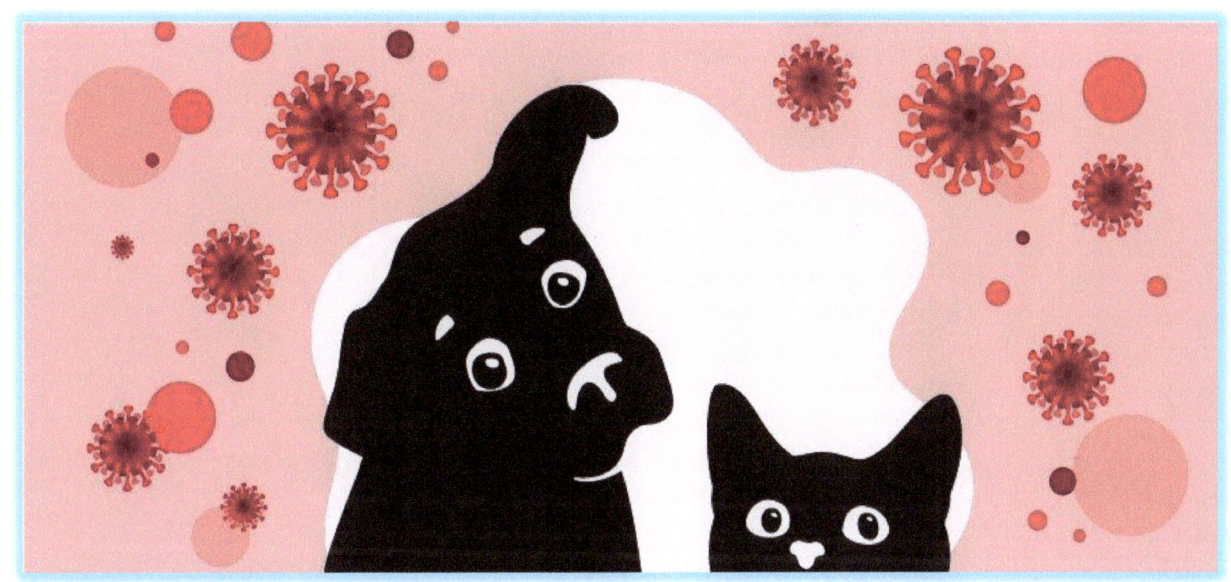

The Coronavirus and Your Pet-A Veterinary Team's Perspective

According to the CDC, some Coronaviruses that infect animals can be spread to humans and then spread between people. One such case has been found and documented in Hong Kung, and recently a very small number of cases were found in the U.S.; however, it is rare. The WHO (World Health Organization) continues to monitor the latest research on this rare occurrence. The safest practice is to protect your pets as you would protect yourselves with social distancing and no more than necessary outside contact.

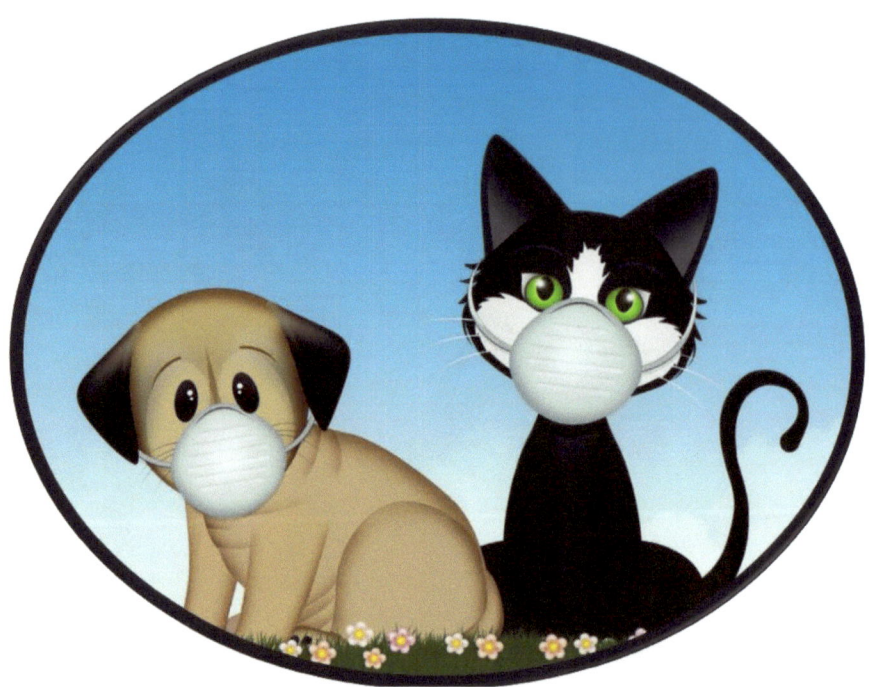

Cats and Dogs-Coronavirus COVID-19 and Our Pets-Best
Bestfriendsvethospital.com

Canine Respiratory Coronavirus

- Shown to cause respiratory disease in dogs
- Referred to as Type 1 CCoV
- First isolated in 2003 in England
  - Found in the lung tissues of affected dogs
  - Similar to strain OC43 of bovine and human coronaviruses
  - Also isolated on European mainland and Japan
  - Dogs in US and Canada have been found to have antibodies

The Coronavirus and your Pet-A Veterinary Team's Perspective

A Note to Parents[1]

The symptoms mentioned previously in children have been linked to COVID-19. It is contagious and is called "Pediatric Multi-System Inflammatory Syndrome." Once a child enters the hospital, they can either test positive for COVID-19 or test negative for COVID-19 but test positive to having coronavirus antibodies. Sometimes children may progress to cardiac arrest and/or kidney failure. Please don't take these symptoms for granted.

Additionally, there are approximately 80 different organs in the human body, and contracting COVID-19 can affect any or all of them in some way that may not be detected immediately. Some known organs that have been affected are:

- lungs, nose, trachea, bronchi, heart
- kidney, bladder, urethra
- skin, pancreas, stomach, liver, brain
- large & small intestine, rectum, anus

Sometimes this virus causes blood clots in the large and/or small blood vessels, which usually leads to stroke-like symptoms in older victims. Some affected individuals have also experienced severe hallucinations. This virus is no joke!

A survey was taken in the early part of July 2020, and the CDC statistics reported the following from the state of Florida,

- of all the cases which tested positive for Coronavirus (SARS-Cop), a third of them were children totaling 23,073;
- 1,213 of those children were hospitalized, and nine of them died.
- 23 of those who tested positive had "Pediatric Multisystem Inflammatory Syndrome" (PMIS), also called "Multisystem Inflammatory Syndrome in Children (MIS-C)."
- Of those 23 cases, 13 were children under the age of 10.

Children over the age of ten can spread this virus at the same rate adults do. Don't be fooled by the rumors going around that children are not seriously affected by COVID-19. The truth is that there simply hasn't been enough research done on children to understand what's going on. Recently (July 2020), 900 cases of COVID-19 had been reported in a daycare center in Texas. Three hundred seven of them were children under 17, and 85 were infants. One hundred forty-seven were hospitalized, and 15 were admitted to intensive care. Three did not make it, and the numbers doubled in the month to follow. *Children are not immune!*

In late July 2020, 338,000 children in the U.S. tested positive for Coronavirus, according to the American Academy of Pediatrics and the Children's Hospital Association survey, which did not include data from Texas or parts of New York, meaning the number of infections is much higher.

In late August 2021, according to CBS News, children now make up 15% of U.S. COVID-19 cases with more and more severe illnesses. The American Academy of Pediatrics reports that 93,824 child COVID-19 cases were ported between July 29, 2021 and August 5, 2021.

As of August 5, 2021, nearly 4.3 million children in the U.S. have tested positive since the start of the pandemic. Health experts believe the Delta Variant (a mutation of COVID-19) is behind the uptick in cases.

As the symptoms with COVID-19 continue to evolve, please seek testing if you or someone you know shows symptoms such as diarrhea, vomiting, or mouth lesions. If a virus test is not available, get tested for the antibodies. At least that will give you something tangible to construct your plan of attack against contracting the virus as well as how to protect yourself and your loved ones from it.

One way to protect kids until our youngest are eligible for the vaccine is to have the people that they're around be vaccinated. Until then, everyone should wear masks—vaccinated and unvaccinated.

Asymptomatic[2] means that you do have the virus and could also be a carrier and spreader of the virus, making others sick, while not feeling sick yourself or having any symptoms whatsoever.

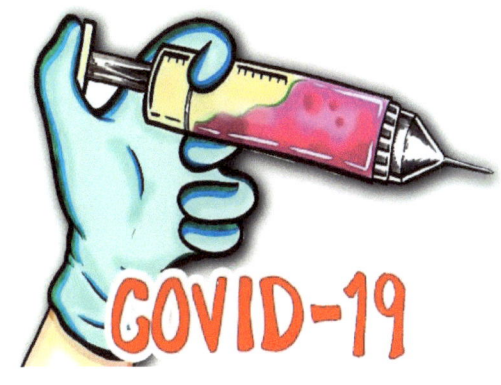

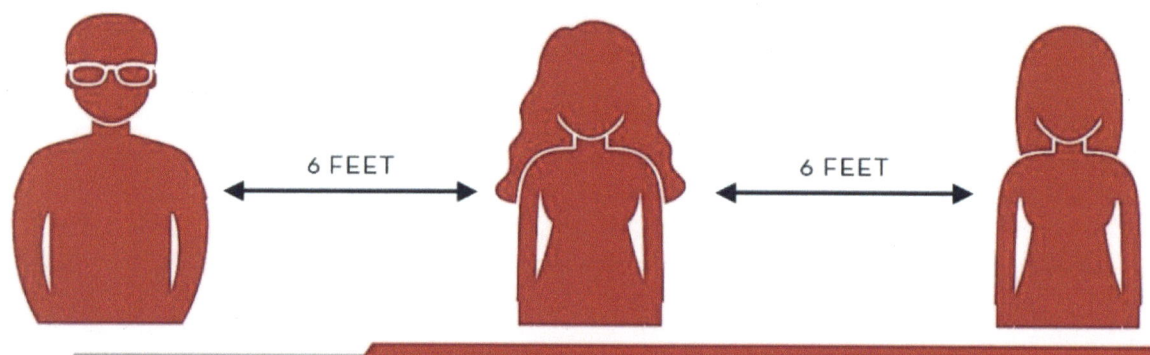

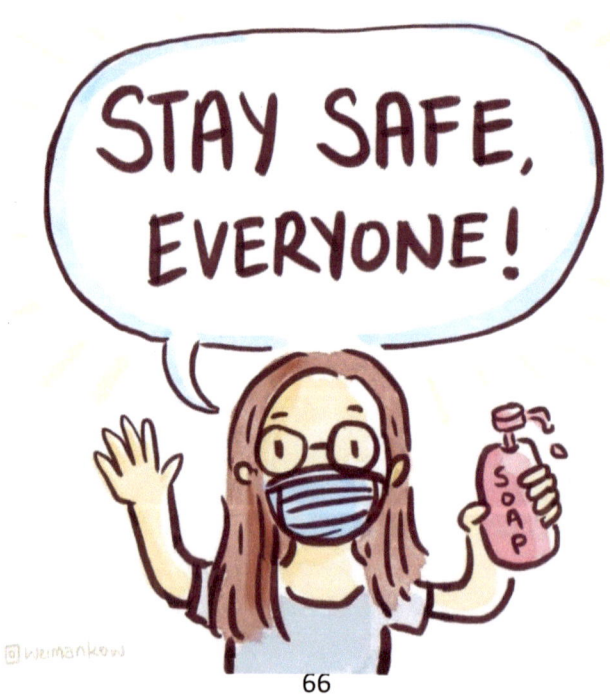

Even though we must be watchful and practical with our safety practices, God has not given us a spirit of fear,

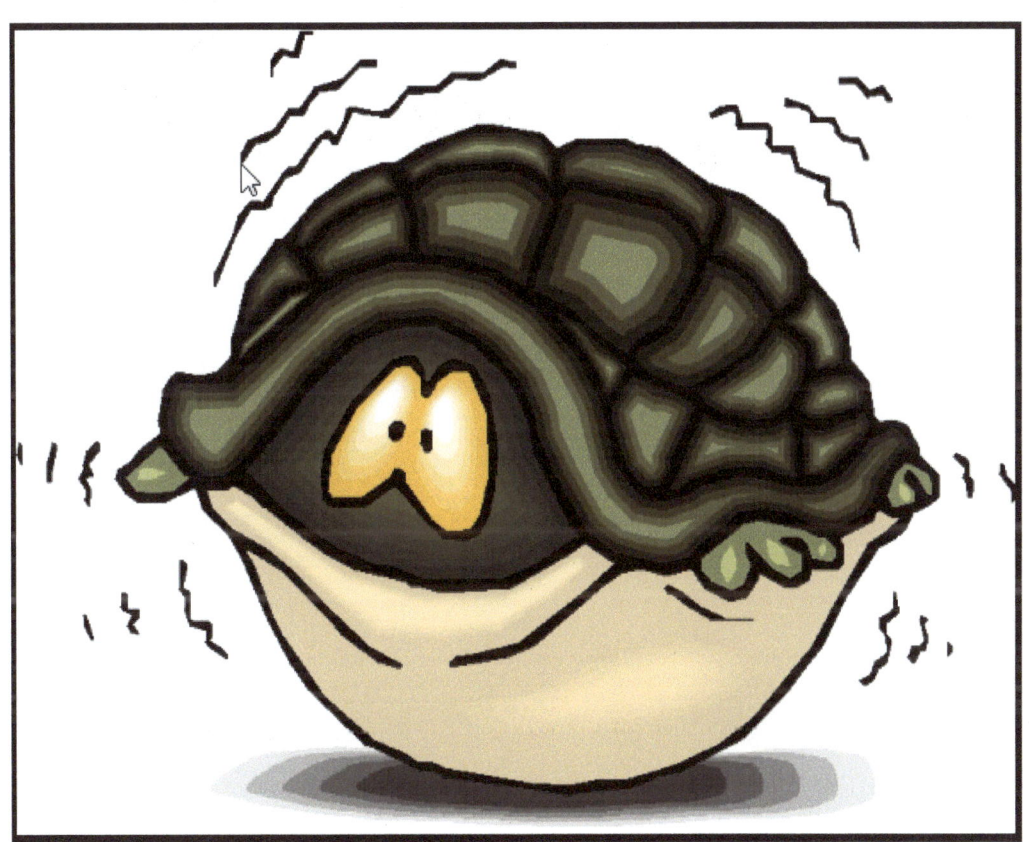

but of power, and love, and a sound mind.

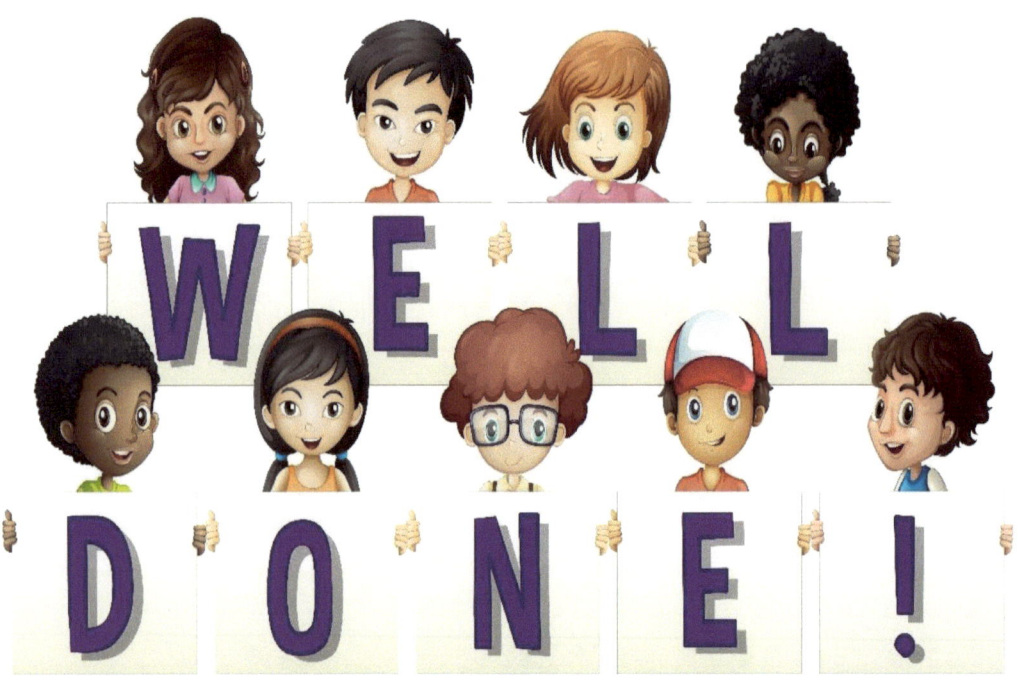

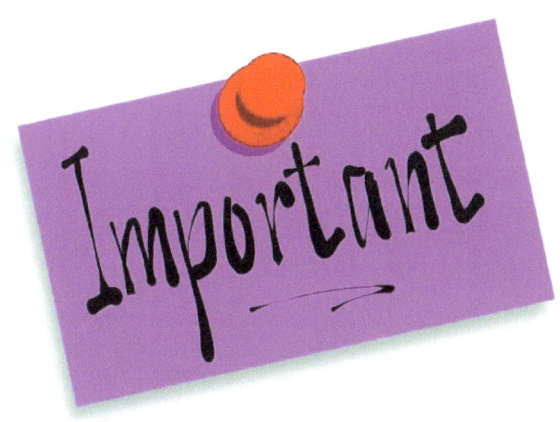

If my people, who are called by my name, will humble themselves and pray and seek my face and turn from their wicked ways, then I will hear from heaven, and I will forgive their sin and will heal their land. 2 Chronicles 7:14 KJV

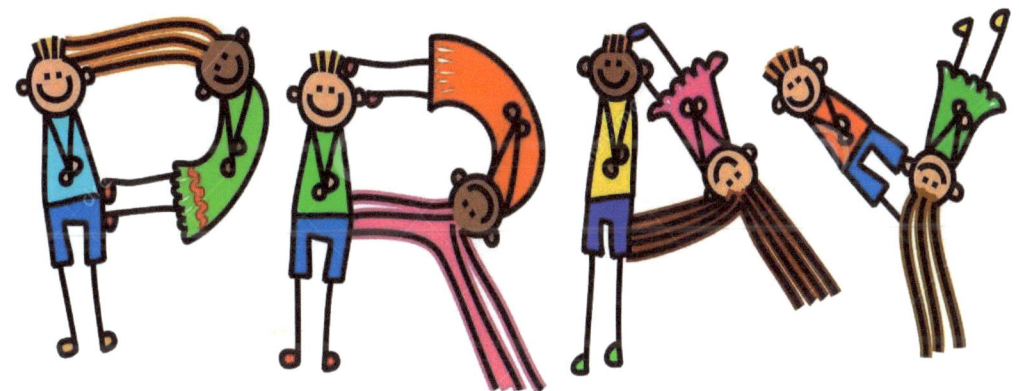

Child Symptoms of COVID-19 Worksheet

Fill in the missing letters here OR copy this page and place your answers there.

__ e __ __ r

I __ __ h __   __ e __   __ y __ __

__ __ s __

S t __ __ a __ __   __ a __ __ s

__ i __ __ r __ e __

V __ m __ __ i __ __

__ k __ __ __   d __ __ c o l __ __ a t __ __ __

S __ __ a __ b __ __ __ y   __ o __ g u __

Child Symptoms of COVID-19 Answer Sheet

Pediatric Multi-Symptom Inflammatory Syndrome

Fever
Itchy Red Eyes
Rash
Stomach Pains
Diarrhea
Vomiting
Skin Discoloration
Strawberry Tongue

Parents, remember that these symptoms can occur up to six weeks after your child has tested negative for Coronavirus but tested positive for Coronavirus antibodies. This means your child contracted the virus somewhere, but you may not have known they had it. This can be a very serious condition leading to dire complications with heart and/or multi-organ failure. New symptoms are popping up daily. You may even need to distance yourself more than six feet apart. Please be watchful and wise in your preventative practices during this period of attacks from an invisible enemy: **COVID-19.**

Other Publications by Linda Mason

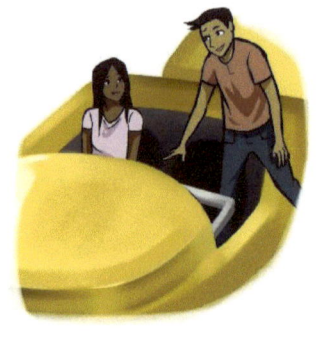

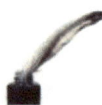

Spirit of Truth Storybook Series from A – Z

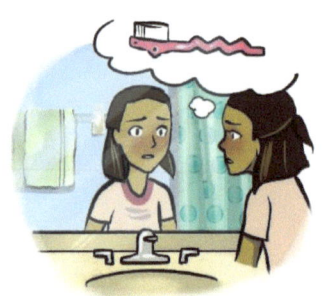

Anxious Arlene
Busy Benny
Catty Carla
Doubtful Denise
Excited Ernesto
Fearless Freddie
Graceful Gregory
Hopeful Henry
Itchy Irvin
Jumping Josey
Kissing Kirkland
Lonely Lucilia
Muddy Maria
Noisy Nelly
Orphaned Ophelia
Pudgy Pete
Quarrelsome Quaniqua
Reckless Ricardo
Shy Stanley

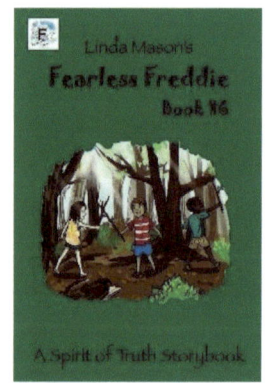

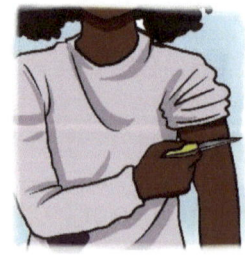

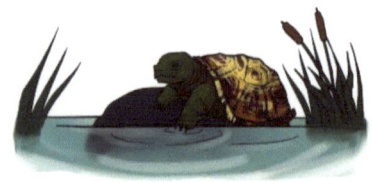

Tearful Tanya
Ungrateful Ursula
Valiant Vivica
Worrying Winston
X-Con Xavier
Yearning Yolanda
Zealous Zeporah

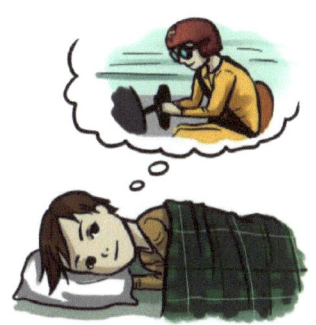

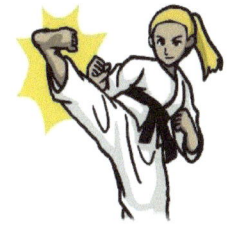

S.O.T. Coloring Book Collection

Anxious Arlene Coloring Book 1
Busy Benny - Fearless Freddie Coloring Book 2
Graceful Gregory - Kissing Kirkland Coloring Book 3
Lonely Lucilia - Pudgy Pete Coloring Book 4
Quarrelsome Quaniqua - Ungrateful Ursula Coloring Book 5
Valiant Vivica - Zealous Zeporah Coloring Book 6

Appetizers from the Word of God ...
Are You Hungry? Volumes 1, 2, & 3

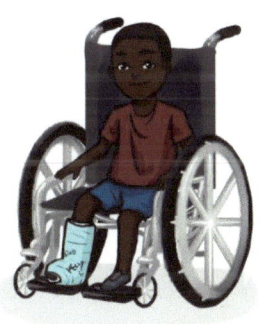

'In His Grace' Project

Beyond Your Control: Book #1
Disappointment Meets Grace: Book #2
Within My Reach: Book #3
Are You Sure About This? Book #4

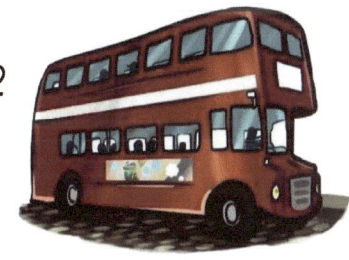

All Grown Up but Still Learning Book #5

Liar! Liar! Pants on Fire! #45
The 'Not-So' Invisible Me
The 'Not So' Invisible Me Chronicles, Volume One
Are Living Beings Really Under the Earth?

BOOK BUNDLES

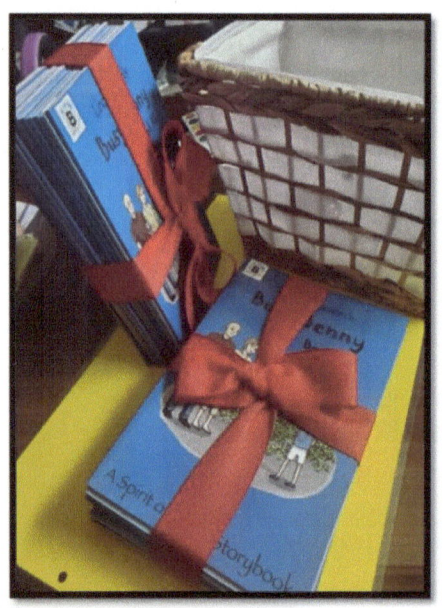
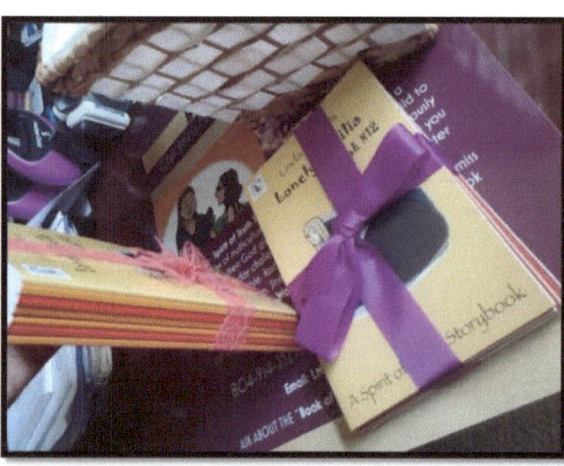
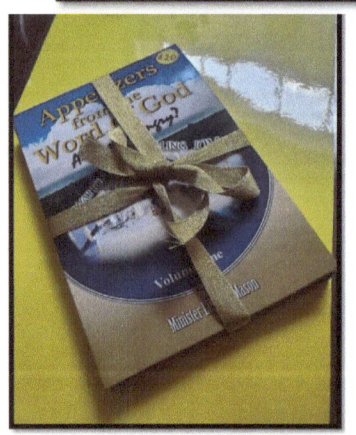
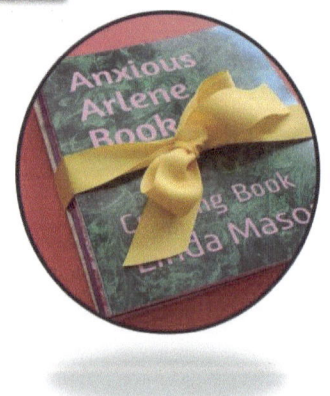
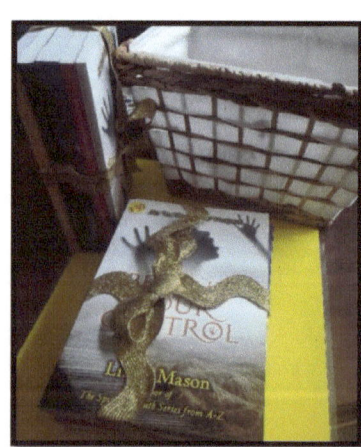

Go to: www.BooksByLMason.com to order

About The Author

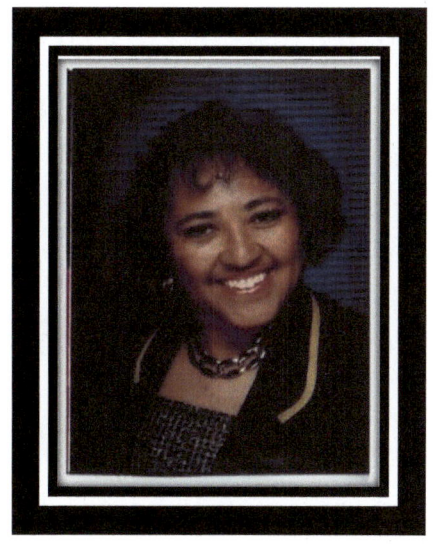

In addition to the *Spirit of Truth Storybook Collection from A-Z,* Linda has published *Appetizers from the Word of God... Are You Hungry?* Volumes 1, 2, & 3 are excellent tools for teaching foundational truths from God's Word in a simplistic manner. She has also published five suspense young adult novels within the series 'In His Grace Project.' Accompanying the SOT Storybook series from A-Z, there are matching coloring books for each story. Four other newly released books entitled 'The Not-So Invisible Me,' a unique children's storybook dealing with youth bullying, 'The Not-So Invisible Me Chronicles, Volume One' (Co-authored with Evelyn P.J. Jefferson), a collaboration of testimonials from other individuals' life experiences, 'Are Living Beings Really Under the Earth?', and a red hot more mature reading level book entitled 'Liar! Liar! Pants on Fire! #45', which is self-explanatory, turned out to be an extremely therapeutic writing project.

    Linda is a native of Suffolk, Virginia, the wife of George B. Mason, Jr., and the mother of three adult children, Tamara, Tiena, and George III. She has three adorable grandchildren, Niyah, Laana, and Aaron. Linda holds an Associate Degree in Early Childhood Education and has a passion for writing. Several of her publications are available in E-book, and some are given away FREE from her website. She plans to have her unique A-Z children's stories available in both English and Spanish and have the 'In His Grace' project paperback and E-Book novels available as audiobooks soon. You may view her progress and take advantage of special 'Bundle' purchases, a FREE storybook download, and expressly many other discounted 'Digital Downloads' at www.BooksByLMason.com.

www.ingramcontent.com/pod-product-compliance
Lightning Source LLC
Chambersburg PA
CBHW040056250526
45473CB00043B/837